# *The Cycle*

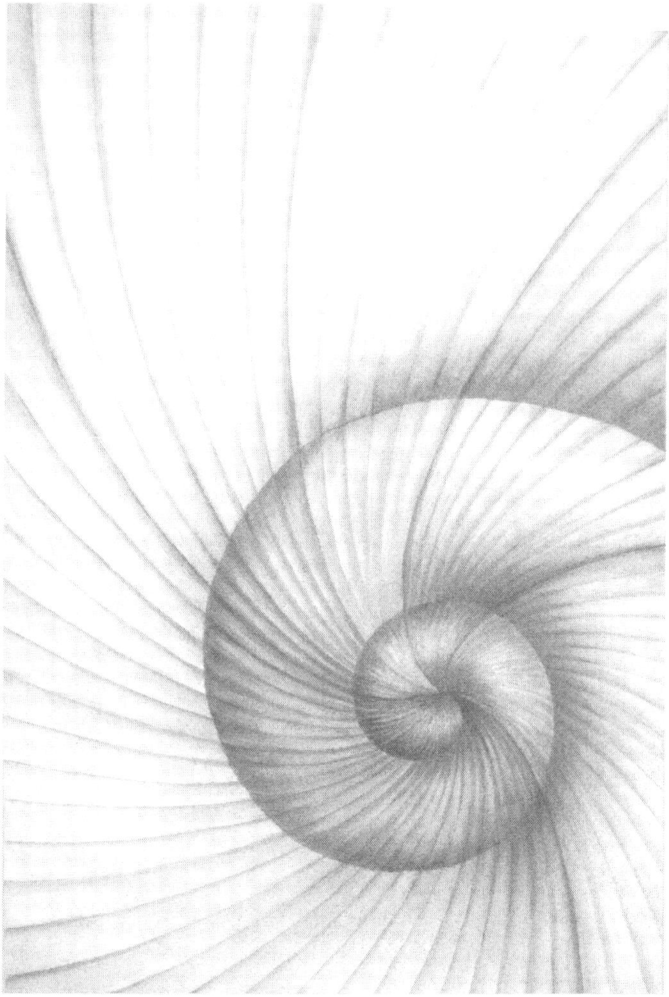

*Creating Smooth Passages
in Every Life Season*

by Pamela Levin

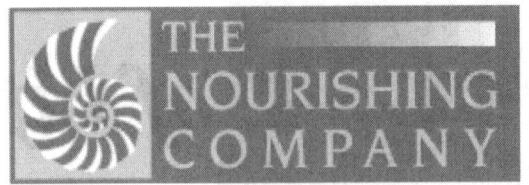

The Nourishing Company
P.O. Box 1429
Ukiah, CA 95482

nourishingcompany.com

**Library of Congress Cataloging-in-Publication Data**
Levin, Pamela.
The Cycle of Life: Creating Smooth Passages in Every Life Season
© 2007 by Pamela Levin
Includes glossary
Printed in the United States of America

No part of this publication may be reproduced, stored in a retrieval system or transmitted in any form or by any means, electronic, mechanical, photocopying, recording or otherwise without the written permission of the publisher.
Portions of this book were published originally in Becoming the Way We Are.

First edition titled Becoming the Way We Are: A Transactional Guide to Personal Development edited by Nora Gallagher, 1974.
Second expanded edition edited by Loni Baur and published by Directed Media, Wenatchee, WA, 1985.
Third edition titled Becoming the Way We Are: An Introduction to Personal Development in Recovery and in Life edited by Marie Stilkind and Paula Clodfelter, published by Health Communications, 1988.
© 1974, 1985, 1988 2007 by Pamela Levin

ISBN 978-0-9672718-3-5
Cover image original by Lee Mothes, Oceans and Dreams studio, www.oceansanddreams.com
Lyrics from "The Circle Game" by Joni Mitchell by permission of Alfred Publishing Co., Inc., Copyright Siquomb Publishing Corporation, MCMLXVI.

*The material in this book is for information purposes only and is not intended as a substitute for medical, psychological or psychiatric treatment or counseling. Do not attempt self—treatment of psychiatric conditions without consulting a qualified health practitioner.*

1. Health. 2. Adulthood. 3. Maturation. 4. Parenting. 5. Interpersonal Relations. 6. Recovery. 7. Self-help.

# *What People Are Saying*

"Now that I know I'm not **supposed** to outgrow what I needed as a child, I can finally feel normal!"
Graphics Designer, California

"I didn't realize there were stages in parenting as well as in the children being raised, and especially that <u>they are the same stages!</u> Fantastic! My parenting skills have now improved and I'm also much more relaxed. Thank you."
Parent, Seattle, Washington

"I found your words very inspiring, and although new concepts to me, very familiar. What I'd been feeling inside was put into words. Thank you."
Twenty—year—old first—time mother, eight months pregnant

"I had trouble getting your books at the school library because, apparently they are always checked out…"
Student, Marin California

"Your book was the perfect healing tool following my divorce. I only wish I'd known before."
Reader, Illinois

"I want to use this information in a class I'm teaching for codependents and adult children of dysfunctional families, and later in a class for nurses, and also on health, healing and wholeness."
RN, Kansas City, Missouri

"Pam Levin's leading—edge work is the foundation for *Homecoming*' Inner Child material and provides the most advanced, effective and compassionate structure available for Inner Child healing."
John Bradshaw, author of *Homecoming*

"To know how you are, read how you were... A beautifully clear exposition of the developmental phases of living."
Alvyn Freed, PhD, author of *TA for Tots, Kids and Teens*

"A useful guide to our stuck points and how to fix them…described in the everyday language of development."
Stephen B. Karpman, MD, author of "Karpman Drama Triangle,"CTM., ITAA

"…adds a new dimension, showing the developmental process of life in T.A. terms."
Dr. L. Jim Anthis, Editor—at—Large, "The Disciple" (Journal of the Christian Church)

"We recommend this book to all our trainees."
Robert Goulding, MD and Mary McClure Goulding, MSW

"We routinely give this book to all new clients to identify developmental issues, to give them a menu for what they might need, and to show them what they might expect in therapy with us."
Jon Weiss, PhD, CTM, ITAA, Empowerment Systems, Littleton, Colorado

"… a valuable must on your reading list. Pam Levin is a pioneer in both theory and practice of Transactional Analysis and is particularly qualified to

share her ideas on how parents' own psychology affects the development of their child. Pam has given us a book which is easy to read and understand but is loaded with solid scientific insights."
Jack Dusay, MD, Past President of International Transactional Analysis Association, author of *Egograms*

"This is a fine summary of how we develop scripts and how we can go beyond them, written from a Transactional Analysis point of view."
Claude Steiner, author of *Scripts People Live* and *Games Alcoholics Play*

"I like Pam and the way she thinks and writes. Both she and her words are clear, direct and encouraging. It's a winning combination."
Muriel James, coauthor of *Born to Win,* Lafayette, California

"This work on development takes Eric Berne's theory and grounds it in health rather than in pathology, thus continuing his tradition of conveying scientific information through a universal language——that of childhood".
Patricia Crossman, LCSW Winner of Eric Berne Memorial Scientific Award

"I use this book in my personal life and I strongly recommend it."
Jean Clarke, author of *Self Esteem: A Family Affair*

"When *Becoming the Way We Are first* came out I used it as a handbook for the therapy I did with clients. Both my clients and I valued it as a resource. Since then, I have only two wellguarded copies remaining which I share with clients in the office. I do not lend them out. This is invaluable core information to healing in psychotherapy."
Jan Elliott LCSW, Ashland, Oregon

# Dedication

To Our Ever—Evolving Inner Self

At every age

In every stage

# Contents

Preface..................................................................................1

**Part One:** NATURE'S GIFT: THE WOMB OF CREATION.............9

**Part Two:** TENDING OUR SEASONS............................................29

   Stage One. ...........................................................................31
     Being: The Ground of Our Existence

   Stage Two. ..........................................................................41
     Doing: The World of Senses and Action

   Stage Three. .......................................................................53
     Thinking: The Conceptual Realm

   Stage Four .........................................................................63
     Identity: Our Ever—Evolving Self

   Stage Five...........................................................................75
     Skillfulness: The "How—To's" of Our Lives

   Stage Six. ...........................................................................87
     Regeneration: Creation and Procreation

   Stage Seven........................................................................97
     Recycling: Manifesting the Promise of Life

**Part Three:** CREATING SMOOTH PASSAGES ............................109
1. Beginning..................................................................113
2. Wisely Meeting Our Need for Recognition ......................123
3. Playing it Straight ......................................................129
4. Authoring Our Own Life Story......................................139
5. Transformation..........................................................147
6. Identifying Self—Sabotage...........................................157
7. Protection .................................................................171
8. Reclaiming Our Essential Selves...................................181
Conclusion: In the End is Our Beginning ..........................187
Resources ......................................................................195
Glossary ........................................................................199
About the Author ...........................................................203
Acknowledgments..........................................................205
Notes ............................................................................207

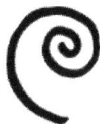

*...turning is...a dance in concert with the galaxies,*

*the molecules and the spiraling form that is*

*the source and essence of the cosmos.*

Coleman Barks

# Preface

These pages are about discovering how we are made, who we really are and how we can work within to transform stress and self—sabotage to support and strength. In short, they are about embracing our own inner life.

When we turn our attention from our outer lives to our inner ones, our condition may be like that of young children who have no way of making sense of what they encounter. Where do we begin? How can we organize? How can we make things work?

That was close to my condition when I met Eric Berne, psychiatrist and founder of Transactional Analysis (TA), at his San Francisco seminars. I sensed that if answers were to be found, this was the place to find them.

Prior to developing TA, Berne's teacher and mentor had been Erik Erickson, a psychiatrist who outlined developmental stages that occur sequentially throughout our lives. At the time I met him, Eric Berne was turning his attention to how we develop what he called "scripts," the unconscious life plans we make in childhood and carry out in adulthood. He was interested in the interactions people have with one another—the transactions—that further the scripts they had chosen for themselves when they were young children. In Transactional Analysis, Berne developed a framework not only for explaining his insights but also for putting those insights at the disposal of laypeople as well as psychiatrists. TA gave people the tools to free themselves from the scripts that held them prisoner. The language of TA was colloquial, and the aim was not long—term adjustment to one's condition but a relatively immediate self—understanding and the consequent choice to change our scripts.

Eric Berne theorized that we make our life's script decisions while we're five and under. I could see the value in studying scripts, but I told him I thought that we had to understand more about how people develop in general to provide the framework for understanding how people develop scripts in particular. Eric, now my teacher and mentor, supported me in following this vein of inquiry, and as I pursued it, I entered into the ongoing conversation about human development, joining Eric Berne, Erik Erickson and Anna Freud, who greatly influenced Erickson, especially in emphasizing that children's emotional symptoms were often related to developmental stages.

Working as a counselor in my own transactional analysis groups in the growth movement of the early 1970s, I noticed that people of the same age shared certain themes and patterns. The 26—year olds were concerned about their connections to others, wanting to join with them, to bond. They were concerned about who they could trust. Meanwhile the 28—year—olds, so close in age to the 26—year—olds, were very different. They related in a contrary, challenging, oppositional

## Preface

way. They wanted "mine" apart from "yours." So striking was this difference between people so close in age, that it piqued my curiosity. I wondered, why should people of the same age but different life circumstances and histories have the same themes and issues in common? Why was this so? I sensed I was seeing one small section of a basic truth which had yet to be revealed.

About this time I moved from the city to a small rural community, where I began to see people's lives within the recurring patterns of nature's rhythms and seasons: nature repeats herself cyclically; why should we be any different? I wondered if the people who shared similar themes were at similar stages of a cycle. With nature as my new teacher and mentor, I began to see the larger pattern I had only glimpsed in my earlier practice. I saw that our lives encompass recurring seasons, each with its own tasks and skills, and that it is our natural design to repeat throughout adulthood the stages we began in childhood.

Returning to the city once again, I shared this knowledge in individual consultations, groups, seminars and workshops. The effect was dramatic. People shed some unnamed inner stress. They calmed down and settled into themselves. They felt better about themselves. They became more friendly and understanding of others. They were coming home to their essential nature.

They wanted to hear this "story of ourselves" again and again. They wanted to explore how it applied to their own lives. Working with people individually and in groups, workshops and seminars, I

## The Cycle of Life

came to understand that our lives evolve in a cycle; that the cycle is composed of stages; that in each stage there are activities—developmental tasks we need to do to evolve successfully; and that the cycle itself offers us guidance for dealing with problem areas and personal pain.

As we worked to discover the origins of the emotional conflicts and personal issues that people brought to these sessions, we found these issues could be deeply rooted, even going back before birth, which is how we discovered that the template for the cycle is actually encoded in the watery world of the womb, before we ever draw our first breath of air.[1]

The implications of these discoveries are far—reaching, affecting every aspect of our lives. The cycle of our lives shapes our sense of self, our internal security and self—confidence, our ability to learn, our friendships, employment, partnering and work life. As we come home to our own cyclic nature and develop effective responses to its challenges, we are able to connect with others in ways that are mutually satisfying and beneficial. We transform our communities as well as ourselves.

It turned out that people far beyond my own groups and workshops were hungry for this information as well. I'd published my discoveries in a slim volume entitled *Becoming the Way We Are*. The first printing sold out in a weekend. The second printing, of 10,000 copies, also sold swiftly. Requests for translations followed, as did subsequent edi-

## Preface

tions and new publishers. *Becoming* was becoming people's personal primer.

Each successive printing brought more letters describing the ways people were using this book in their lives. They were applying it in classrooms, boardrooms and bedrooms. They were using it to aid addiction recovery, to assist the mentally or physically challenged, to help seniors complete end—of—life issues. They were parents and grandparents, teachers of preschool, grade school, and high school. College instructors made it an assigned text in child development, psychology and family life courses. Therapists, pastoral counselors and organizational consultants made it a central reference in their work. Graduate students made it the foundation for their theses. *Becoming* dovetailed with neurological repatterning work being carried out with people experiencing brain dysfunctions. It spawned a children's book in the Flemish language,[2] was used to develop a parenting system,[3] inspired a company making products using the material,[4] and provided the foundation for the developmental and Inner Child material in the New York Times bestseller *Homecoming*.[5] From the University of Quebec in Canada came a request to translate this material into French, saying Amerindian students were demanding a French edition, as they recognized the cycle and its stages as their Medicine Wheel.[6]

This was indeed a phenomenal reception. Why did it strike such a chord?

Certainly, having one's private, often unnamed, inner life outlined on paper as common to all can be a powerful experience.

## The Cycle of Life

But to discover a quality of our essential nature, and to recognize that this very nature invites us ceaselessly and cyclically to become more fully ourselves, is to discover a map for navigating our inner lives. It is to realize that we all have emotional brains that do not work according to the same principles as those of our logical or thinking brains. Having this fact laid bare in black and white is an enormous comfort when we had thought there was something wrong with us because our lives are not unfolding in a logical and linear way.

This information also strikes a resonant chord in us because it is about the story of ourselves collectively. As each of us individually comes home to the cyclic unfolding of our own personal, *inner* lives, we reveal the common patterns we each share with every other. This is very different from the stories of ourselves we are used to hearing, ones derived from studying *outer* manifestations of our lives, that is, those behaviors, qualities or achievements that can be measured, quantified or observed.

The critical role of our emotional brains and our hunger to know more about them was recently demonstrated by the success of Daniel Goleman's *Emotional Intelligence* and *Social Intelligence.* Like the themes in *Becoming the Way We Are,* these books underscored that we have inner lives in the first place, that our inner lives have everything to do with actual physical brain and body structures and are not a function of our imagination or our pathology, and that these inner processes which produce our EQ are far more significant determinants of our successes or failures in life than our IQ. The enthusiastic reception

## Preface

and immediate application of these messages demonstrated how hungry we are to know how we are made and how we can manage these aspects of our lives. Indeed, it is through our inner developmental process that we learn "people" skills——those "soft" facilities that are the key to having relationships that work, that are satisfying and mutually beneficial. We develop based on our inner nature, but *what* we learn——even *whether* we learn is a result of the interactions that take place between ourselves and others. Our lives follow an inborn code as they unfold, and as they do, we engage in an interactional learning process.

Probably nowhere are the resources we have developed more called upon or more exposed than in the process of rearing children. When we parents come home to our own inner design, we discover that we repeat the same stages our children are growing through. When we apply what we are learning about the stages and tasks of our own inner cycle to our children, we improve our parenting skills and our own lives at the same time. We find that that our children learn to respect themselves as they are actually made, and also to respect others as they are actually made, for their needs and others' are the same. This prevents a great deal of risky behavior, without stifling children's independence. In fact, the extent to which a culture is healthy is the extent to which it supports this fundamental and universal pattern in all of its members in all of their ages.

The message is clear from the explorers of the inner world whose experiences, when shared, reveal the pattern described in these pages:

## The Cycle of Life

The more we become free of the constraints of trying to make ourselves be other than the way we are made, the more we live in our basic nature, free to grow and evolve as the process takes us, stage by stage, through this progression of life. It is at once a message not only of hope but of success, of growth and of healing, speaking as it does to our essential human nature, so hungry to be validated in this modern world which often casts it aside.

This book, which includes material from the original publication of *Becoming the Way We Are*, is dedicated to that process. Part One describes this cyclic blueprint and its stages, mapping the life journey that we each travel individually; yet share with every other human being.

Part Two presents individually each life season within the cycle, including its childhood beginnings, its manifestations in our adult lives, and what we need to do to complete a successful passage in each.

Part Three outlines the process of embracing the teachings offered by the cycle. It introduces some ways to move from resisting inner discoveries to accepting them as invitations to become more conscious and free.

Together they provide an introduction to and an overview of the process of turning our usual, outward focus to an inward one of coming back home. Still, it is a map of the route, not the route itself. We who read the symbols must understand that words can only represent and not replace the spirit, which is what we each provide.

# PART ONE

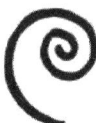

# NATURE'S GIFT
## The Womb of Creation

*For those who seek understanding, the circle is their mirror... it is the lodge of our bodies, our minds and our hearts. It is the cycle of all things that exist. The circle is our way of touching and of experiencing harmony with every other living thing around us.*

Hyemeyohsts Storm
Plains Indian spiritual elder

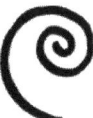

Everywhere we look we see that nature's pattern of growth is cyclic. Plants sprout, flower, go to seed, become compost, sprout again, and slowly plant species evolve. Animal species follow a similar pattern, with traits passing through generations and reshaping the animals themselves. All that we know of nature follows a cyclic pattern: the ebb and flow of the tides, the waxing and waning moon in a month, the months in a season, the seasons of the year, the orbits of planets, the spiraling of galaxies—all of these cycles demonstrate this truth.[7]

As part of nature, why should we be any different? Why should we be the only beings who do not also pass through repeating seasons or stages in the course of our lives? Why should we think that the architecture of our own lives is different from everything else that exists in nature? What if we are each our own spiral galaxy in miniature? What if our lives revolve around an inner orbit, periodically returning to the place we started?

Or, to move from the cosmic to the comic, what if life truly is "not one thing after another, but the same thing over and over"? Beginning a new job or moving to a new city, we again feel the world is as new as do newborns, however graceful we've become, however easily we laugh at ourselves. Challenged by the stubbornness of a recalcitrant child, we can find ourselves succumbing to a power struggle, no matter how mature we've become. We reach certain ages and find that our friends feel restless in the same ways at those ages, or feel the same hopefulness. When we look for patterns in our lives, we become aware of not only the repetition of certain themes and issues over time but also the regularity of their recurrence. And when we compare these regular, recurring patterns in our lives with the patterns recurring in the lives of others, their commonality is a revelation.

Recurring themes in our lives fascinate us because they echo something deep within us and don't fit our linear model of life. We usually think of our lives as a progression or journey from "point a" to "point z." The starting and stopping points could be birth and death, or immaturity and wisdom, or innocence and experience, and we might envision our path itself as "the straight and narrow" way or as a meandering trail marked by sidetracks and cul—de—sacs, but the metaphor we use is linear. We expect our lives to unfold in a series of stages or "times of life" that we leave behind as we pass through them. So when we find elements of those former times in our current time of life, we are intrigued.

Our linear model of life has an immediate basis in reality: we observe one another grow from birth through maturity to death in a linear progression. All parents are familiar with the milestones of their children's physical developmental sequence: babies lift their heads, roll over, sit up, crawl, cruise, walk. Parents might be less familiar with

# PART ONE

the subtler developmental markers, such as the baby's being able to keep an image of Mom in mind when Mom is out of the room, or a child's understanding that a cup of water in a tall narrow glass and a cup of water in a short wide glass is the same amount of water. These subtler markers indicate developmental stages in children's thinking, and other markers document stages in children's emotional development.

From infancy to adulthood, we change so radically in so many ways that the changes are hard to miss. After we move into adulthood, however, changes that we can observe from the outside become less obvious. Our bodies change far more slowly than they did in childhood, and our interior lives don't add new abilities as much as they deepen abilities already there. "Deepen," "enrich," and "add dimension to" are ways that we talk about the growth that happens in adulthood. Over the decades leading to old age, rather than continue our childhood developmental trajectory of adding whole new capacities to our bodies and intellects and psyches, we gather experience and somehow (we hope) become wise.

The idea that our development continues into adulthood has remained an open conversation among researchers. Many agree that we do indeed undergo stages of development after we reach adulthood, but there is less consensus about the specific stages, their tasks, and their timing. In popular culture, too, there is a lot of variation in the ways we think about the tasks and challenges of adulthood. We are familiar with the notion of a midlife crisis, for example, but when is mid—life? Is it 35? 40? 50? What does "midlife" mean, and does its timing differ from person to person?

One reason for the disparity among ways of looking at the timing and tasks in adult development is the linear model itself. If we expect adult development to continue along the same lines as childhood development, we look for developmental markers of some sort showing up in similar ways in all people's lives, like the milestones of childhood. But adult development doesn't have the simplicity of childhood development. In childhood, each stage of development creates new "blocks" that the child uses to lay a foundation of physical, cognitive, and emotional skills and capacities. Adult development doesn't create new blocks——it builds on that foundation. To put it another way, our task as adults is to add depth and dimension to the skills, capacities, and understanding that we first developed in childhood. We do this by revisiting the developmental stages of childhood. The developmental stages of adult life, then, are the recurring stages of childhood development.

The linear model of our lives, which does indeed capture the foundation—laying progression of childhood development, cannot adequately describe the experience of adults. The tasks we face as adults are not by their nature new to us; they are more sophisticated versions of challenges we have met already in childhood. Handling authority, discovering boundaries, finding our place in a group——tasks like these have a familiar childhood core, however grown up the circumstances and details. Our experience of these tasks, our feelings when

## Part One

we are living with them, and the ways we choose to meet and carry out these tasks create a pattern of recurring themes in our lives. When we look closely at these patterns, and compare our lives' patterns with the lives of others, we begin to see commonalities in timing. We begin to see that the developmental stages of childhood recur in a predictable cycle throughout adulthood. That short line that described our childhood sequence of development repeats itself, turning back to the beginning to run through the stages in order. Over time, the line becomes a spiral.

Once we see this cycle at work in our lives, we begin to notice references to recurring cycles everywhere. The range of cultural references demonstrates the symbol's universality: the earliest Chinese ideograms used the spiral to depict "return" or "homecoming," and the spiral has the same meaning for Native American Hopi; painted on the walls of houses in Tibet, it means "home, the place one returns to."[8] Whether we turn our attention to the coils of the tiny molecules of our DNA, which is aptly described as a spiral staircase, to the charged nodes of the planet earth, [9] or to the immensity of our Milky Way galaxy, we find this same spiral pattern.[10]

"Cycles are meaningful," Edward R. Dewey tells us, "and all science that has been developed in the absence of cycle knowledge is inadequate and partial. . . . any theory of economics, sociology, history, medicine or climatology that ignores non—chance rhythms is as manifestly incomplete as medicine was before the discovery of germs."[11] Cycles are the elegant, self—replicating blueprint of our inner lives.[12]

## The Cycle of Life

Our own inner blueprint begins with the foundation—laying developmental sequence of our childhood. This sequence presents us with a model of our complete cycle, comprised of six stages, each with its own tasks necessary to emotional, cognitive, and physical development. The stages present themselves readily to us, with their obvious developmental markers; human beings have developed through exactly these stages in every generation, in every civilization, for as long as humans have been human. We may feel that we've discovered something new in realizing that the six stages repeat themselves cyclically as we mature, until we remember that 5000 years ago, the *I Ching* (*Book of Changes*) described the basic pattern of growth, or change, in life as having six stages, with the seventh bringing return.

The childhood cycle begins at birth and runs through all six stages from birth to age thirteen. Then the layering of cycles continues. At a purely chronological level, we come back to the beginning phase of the cycle and undergo a complete repetition. This happens every thirteen years throughout our lives. This recurrence seems to be biologically determined, and is not subject to alteration, regardless of life events or our attitude towards it.

But sheer chronological or biological recurrence is not the only way that we undergo the cyclic pattern we experienced in childhood. A second way we enter cycles is harmonic: we repeat a stage because we are interacting closely with some person at a different stage and therefore resonate with his or her stage. Becoming a parent at age twenty—eight, say, our biological cycle is repeating our two—year—old stage,

## Part One

but we also start the beginning of a new cycle in harmony
fant.

Yet a third way of entering a cycle results from being triggered by life events, which have cycles of their own. If we are in Stage Four, for example, when a parent dies, we are triggered back to Stage One, beginning a cycle of grieving in addition to our biological stage. Or we might be in a biological repetition of Stage Five, for example, actively building and updating our skills on a new level when we marry, which triggers the beginning of an additional cycle relative to the marriage.

These different ways of entering a cycle mean that we can be in several different stages at one time, depending on our focus. This resonates with our experience of life: we can be calm and skillful at work, playful and physical with our baby, contrary on the phone with a sibling, and focus on enforcing boundaries with our partner in a conversation about housekeeping. All in one day. The layers of cycles that we experience make it possible for us to deepen our foundational skills and capacities. This is our developmental task as a grownup. This is the movement toward wisdom.

We enter a relationship and begin a cycle that spans its course. We become parents and start a shared cycle with our child. We enter a room, attend a meeting, and leave, having experienced the cycle in miniature. In other words, because this cycle is a basic component of our make—up, we experience it as a fundamental organizing principle in every part of our lives, from the smallest through the largest. Cycles are so natural to our experience that we commonly use them to describe our lives poetically, as does Joni Mitchell in the lyrics to her song, "The Circle Game":

*We're captives on a carousel of time.*
*We can't return, we can only look*
*Behind from where we came*
*And go round and round and round*
*In the circle game.*[13]

The layers of harmonic cycles, with event—triggered cycles occurring in addition to our biologic repetition, form the same pattern British physicist Lewis F. Richardson observed and elaborated so poetically in his attempts to analyze and accurately predict the weather:

*Big whorls have little whorls*
*Which feed on their velocity*
*And little whorls have lesser whorls*
*And so on to viscosity.*[14]

But cycles are not merely poetic descriptions of our lives. Just as science supports Richardson's description of weather patterns as whorls, so does science reveal our development to occur in recurring cycles. Nevertheless, our returns through the stages we began in childhood, although entirely natural, may seem abnormal to us for a number of reasons. First, given the apparent randomness and variety of

## PART ONE

our experiences on the surface of life, discovering this order may be surprising. Next, we may be accustomed to thinking about life as a linear progression in which there is no return. We may have been expected to "put away the things of childhood" and thus have been prevented from experiencing as adults our continuing childlike nature in the unending repetition of stages.

Further, we may have attempted to deal with the limitations we endured in earlier stages by refusing to allow ourselves to experience or remember much of our childhood. Ineffective as it may have been, it was one way to cope.

And even when we notice that elements in our lives repeat themselves, if we are not able to grow and heal with each opened door, we may feel saddened and hopeless.

Recycling through the stages offers us a better alternative. We can accept the cyclic nature of our journey through life, thus ending a war with our own nature. We can take care of our own internal business, actively engaging in our own unfolding life process by carrying out the tasks presented to us in each stage of the cycle.

### The Six Stages of the Cycle

The cyclical evolution of our lives means that we return to certain issues and themes over the course of our lives as we pass, and return to pass again, through these same six fundamental stages:

Stage One: Being: The Ground of Our Existence

# The Cycle of Life

Stage Two:Doing: The World of Senses and Action
Stage Three:Thinking: The Conceptual Realm
Stage Four:Identity: Our Ever—Evolving Self
Stage Five:Skillfulness: The How—to's of Our Lives
Stage Six:Regeneration: The Ability to Create and Procreate
Stage Seven:Recycling: Manifesting the Promise of Life

As we pass through each stage in childhood, we become familiar with this developmental design. We begin to develop its basic powers and abilities and lay the groundwork for how we will repeat the stages in the future.

As we repeat the stages in adulthood, we have naturally recurring opportunities to continue to develop emotionally, by carrying out developmental tasks associated with each stage. This is how we can refine, update and further expand each aspect of our selves, and in doing so, align ourselves with the cyclic process of nature and claim the capacities that are inherently ours.

We may feel this as an individual, private, inner process, but all of us move through this interior developmental cycle in the same way, just as we all moved through the physical developmental stages of babyhood in the same sequence. Our interior cycle also reflects basic cosmic laws, since each stage exists in a harmonious, proportional relationship to the others. In other words, the length of each stage exists in proportion to every other: the first stage is six months long, the next stage is twice that length, and the third stage is the length of stages one and two combined, and so forth. The lengths of the stages relative to one another did not seem significant at first——especially because people working on their cycle focused on the tasks necessary in each stage——but working with the stages over time revealed that the lengths of the stages relative to one another reflect the classical "golden proportion" Euclid described over two thousand years ago.[15] Also called the "Golden Ratio" or the "Divine Proportion," it was considered one of the natural architectural or design laws, since all of nature——the structure of a leaf, the dimensions of a horse——fit this ratio. Egyptians built the pyramids according to these proportions. We know Leonardo da Vinci's drawing of a human form inside a circle as a demonstration of the proportions of the human body, but we know this particular drawing because Leonardo drew it; all of the Renaissance painters would have made a sketch like that to keep their figure studies accurate. The golden proportion was the basic proportion of life.[16]

That the golden proportion applies to our recurring cycle of growth makes perfect sense. Why shouldn't our interior design reflect the same proportions as our exterior? Our interior design's cyclic code is composed of this repeating series of six stages, with the seventh bringing return to the first stage. These stages are time—tagged teachable moments: a door opens to an opportunity for essential life learning, stays open for a pre—established period of time, and then closes. During our prenatal life and childhood, we are creating fundamental programming that will serve or sabotage us our entire lives. Our time—

tagged unfolding process continues into adulthood, when we have opportunities to learn more sophisticated aspects of the lessons presented during foundational stages. These adult repetitions, based as they are on foundational layers, can activate those layers and any unfinished business that may lie there. Why is this so?

Many reptiles and lower mammals are born with rote behaviors "hard—wired" into their brains. As human beings, we have hard—wired reflexes too. But we are also able to adapt our responses to a situation based on what we've learned previously. In other words, we are both hard—wired and "soft—wired." An example of our inborn hard— wiring is the system that allows us to automatically send all our bodily resources to fight, freeze, or flee in the presence of danger. But because we're also soft—wired, we can make decisions based on our storehouse of experiences: we can remember what happened when we encountered a particular sign of danger before, or can apply something we've learned in one situation to one with similar components, say, and choose ways to handle the current challenge in totally new ways.

We humans acquire the programming that is inborn in other animals over the course of our prenatal and childhood stages, filling out our genetic programming——the hard wiring——with what we have learned so that our system can handle a variety of tasks automatically. The long learning period we have in relation to other mammals is necessary because we have to acquire learning that is innate in other species. We gain this knowledge by consciously participating in an experience, then relegating what we've learned to our collection of

PART ONE

automatic responses. Because those automatic skills were learned, not programmed genetically, they are "extra—genetic programming." For example, as toddlers we find out that when we drop something, it falls. Originally this is fascinating news. Only later will we understand the concept of gravity.

As newborns, we don't know how to blink when something comes too close to our eyes, but once learned the behavior becomes automatic. We learn how to take in nourishment by sucking and swallowing, which once learned becomes routine. We find out how to calm ourselves when feeling anxious as we receive help from our caregivers, developing a repertoire of ways to restore our equilibrium. Neurosociology has shown that the part of our brains that lights up when we are nurtured as a baby does the same when we as adults use an effective strategy to calm anxiety.

Much learning occurs only during time—tagged teachable moments: something must be learned during a certain time, such as an infant's ability to suck. When a baby sucks, it is learning to take in things it needs for survival. This is a time—tagged skill. If the baby has a cleft palate and is unable to suck, for example, gaining its sustenance instead from tube feedings during its first several months, then the teachable moment is gone and the skill remains unlearned, for the next time—tagged skill is now presented.

This extra—genetic system is how we attain the behavioral foundation that is pre—wired into other species.[17] We are pre—wired to learn, and that learning itself becomes an extension of our brains' programming, enabling us to blaze new behavioral and cultural pathways on short time scales, and thus greatly enhancing our chances of survival as individuals and also as a species.[18]

The model for this extra—genetic system is the same as that built from our inborn, hard—wired system——our DNA. Our extra—genetic programming is composed of six parts with the last, like our DNA's programming, being "Repeat yourself similarly." We grow through the six stages and follow the last instruction, to repeat similarly, thus replicating the same pattern our DNA uses to replicate inside our cells. Not surprisingly, it is a process that also parallels the six days of creation referred to in Genesis.[19]

None of this crucial development takes place in isolation. It is, in fact, transactional——that is, our development forms through our experiences in transactions or *exchanges* with others. As we grow through childhood, we weave together the strands of our extra—genetic learning system from three key ingredients: from the developmental tasks we carry out at the stage we are in, from the responses of our environment (primarily from parents or caregivers) to those tasks, and from the bond that connects the child who is learning and the grownups who are the caregivers. In this way we replicate the model of our own cellular DNA, weaving together the strands of nature and nurture.

We learn "people skills" as our inner developmental process unfolds. These are "soft" faculties——the keys to having relationships that work, that are satisfying and mutually beneficial. Our development itself occurs sequentially, with "windows of opportunity" opening at specific times to enable us to learn particular skills, but *what* we learn——even *whether* we learn——is a result of the interactions that take place between ourselves and others. In other words, our lives unfold via an inborn cyclic code from which we engage in an interactional learning process.

The complete picture of this code and its construction was originally uncovered with the tools of Transactional Analysis, which are used to discover what goes on between people. A composite of the experiences of many people was then constructed. Recently social neuroscience has been able to validate this extra—genetic programming process. Brain imaging has shown that mirror neurons fire in one person, mapping what goes on in the brain of another, making the behavior of another downloadable. In this way the emotional state of others is indeed contagious.[20]

Once we establish our internal learning system, we are likely to reflect its contents in our outer world unless we consciously decide otherwise. That's because we call forth automatic responses from our extra—genetic library for how to read other people's cues, how to listen, how to pay attention and to act in social situations, and so forth. In this way, the contents of our extra—genetic system can preordain both our interpretations of reality and our responses to it, thus reproducing in our outer world what is contained in our inner one.

In addition, our extra—genetic system can contain codes that are in violation of our genetic codes and therefore reduce the biological integrity of our physical/emotional system in some way. The dysfunctional aspects of this system as they appear in adulthood are called a "script" (a life plan made in childhood, now unconscious), which is addressed in Part Three.[21]

The next section, Part Two, presents each stage or season of the cycle separately, with a short description, a summary listing common components, and a set of activities so we can understand not only that particular stage but also how we experience it personally. By answering the questions in each section, we are participating actively in learning about our stages. By applying these ideas to our own lives, we more fully understand the attributes of each stage of the cycle, discover what we need to do to grow and evolve in healthy ways, and learn how to relate to other people who are in this stage. Each section includes ways we can promote our own and others' emotional growth plus descriptions of what we need for a smooth passage.

Before going on——a word about the categories within the stages. Ego states are named in each stage, totaling six ego states. Readers familiar with transactional analysis are used to thinking of three ego states (Parent, Adult and Child); these are the ones that are easily identified in the transacting adult. Sub—parts of these develop during the initial stages of childhood, and an integrating "skin" is added during adolescence. The following section includes six stages, each with its own part of our ego because these subparts develop during the earlier stages.

## PART ONE

Interactions that we have with others are called "transactions." The type of transactions we have that include an ulterior motive, a switch and a payoff are called games. Various games were elaborated initially in Eric Berne's *Games People Play*. Their connection to each of the stages is described in my own *Cycles of Power*.

Injunctions are parental messages we incorporated and are still using to program our present lives. For example, the injunction "Don't exist" may be carried out by working hard and then acting out in a self—destructive, reckless manner, or by smoking or allowing ourselves to be around situations or people that are not safe.

The reader need not have previous experience with transactional analysis to use this book since terminology and concepts are defined as they come up. TA's laypeople—friendly approach has remained clear and helpful over more than four decades. In this book it empowers us to walk through the doors that our recurring cycle of life opens for us.

And so, on to discover the stages, one by one.

# PART TWO

## Tending Our Seasons

*To everything there is a season, and
a time to every purpose under heaven.*

Ecclesiastes 3:1

# STAGE ONE

BEING

## The Ground of Our Existence

*(Birth to Six Months)*

*Never lose a holy curiosity.*

Albert Einstein

The events of the first six months of our lives are crucial to all the rest of our development. The way we experience our existence for the rest of our lives is largely determined by the foundation laid down while we are still helpless. Our first basic "set," internal working model, or extra—genetic program is the building block upon which we support all our later developmental experiences and decisions. It is our basic position in life, our okay—ness, and the basis of how we relate to our right to exist. It is our basic existential position.

All the experiences from which we derive our first program are recorded in an ego state called our Natural Child. They are on film and on file in each of us, a personal documentary of how we each arrived at our basic life position. They are represented in our dreams by floating—feeling—formless—misty images that may be filled with highly pleasurable sensations or ghouls, monsters, sadistic attackers and unknown dangers, depending upon our early life experiences.

During our first months we are completely helpless physically. We can only kick and flail aimlessly, except for one purposeful behavior——our ability to cry. Crying is the first stimulus we create outside the womb, our first attempt to communicate with the rest of the world. It is our first ability to be adequate. The responses of the environment to our cry complete our first transactions.

Our relationship to our environment is our umbilical cord to life because we are not capable of thinking or carrying out complicated tasks. We depend on borrowing these capacities from others through a relationship called symbiosis. Transactionally, a symbiotic relationship is one in which the functions of feeling, thinking and doing are shared between two or more people. Our first program is the result of our transactions in this relationship.

We reach conclusions about what life is like based on transactions around two basic needs: feeding and stroking. Taking in food, we stimulate and define our innermost physical boundary or gut. Taking in physical strokes through touch, we define our outermost boundary or skin. In addition to supplying fuel for a rapidly growing body, in meeting these needs we experience that we exist physically and that we are real. We also discover where our own body stops and the rest of the world begins.

If we are required to wait time after time when we signal that our fuel supply is low, we may decide that our existence is not important, or that we are not to be trusted about communicating and fulfilling our needs. Later we may not recognize that we need something until our blood sugar is dangerously low, or our spinal nerves are vibrating with pain. Conversely, if the grownups taking care of us were overanxious, they may have anticipated what we needed, thereby preventing us from developing the capacity to organize the sea of sensations in our bodies in such a way that we can *know* that we need something, let alone know *what* we need. If early experiences were painful, we may act powerful, strong, angry, hard and cold as adults as a way of protecting our scared, hungry, needy baby feelings.

When we repeat this Being stage in adult life, we need to carry out the same tasks we did as infants, but on a different level. Like infants, we need to *be* rather than *do.* We need to take this opportunity to gradually become more present in our lives——particularly with regard to how we sustain ourselves. At this time we are preoccupied with the connections with others that sustain us. We are taking in, filling up; in fact, it's likely that we want to eat frequently. We have a short attention span. We are establishing answers to such queries as: "Is it OK for me to be here?" "Are my needs OK?" "Who do I feel safe with?" "Who do I feel threatened by?" "Who is it OK to connect to?" "What relationships sustain me?" "Who can I trust, and in what way?" "Who do I distrust?"

These developmental tasks address the "soft wiring" in the same part of our brains that handled our reflex activity as infants: our medulla and cord. The descending neurons in this part of our brains play a significant role in regulating postural muscle tone.

In our relationships with others, we simply want to "be" rather than do. We like to slow down and tune in with them. We enjoy being in the presence of those who nourish and sustain us. We need to express our true feelings and emotional needs to them. We want to be physically close and often touching. We absorb their presence, joining with them, almost as if we are part of the same person. And we love being fed in various ways, having food prepared or provided for us or even affectionately popped in our mouths.

If we are unwilling to take opportunities for "being" time as adults, that may point to such early life decisions as: "I'm OK, valuable, only as long as I'm doing something; I'm not OK just being me," or "My feelings and emotional needs are not OK," or "I don't have the right to exist."

In the process of finishing emotional business from our Being stage, we are greatly aided by those who exude a nurturing, supportive and affectionate presence. Whether by their words, actions or both, they convey to us support of our right to *be*. They attune with our feelings and demonstrate that they compassionately receive and understand our emotional selves. As we take in their care and encouragement we are using new, real, healthy Being experiences to gradually reprogram the neurological patterning we put in place as infants——patterns which control the physical reflexes of our sustaining systems. As we learn to share what we are feeling and needing, and as we have those communications received and understood without judgments or blame, we undergo the new emotional Being experiences that we need in order to change our original, limiting decisions and create a new life position. Now we can be glad we are alive. We can choose to experience the truth——that we are indeed a Child of the universe and have a right to be here.

## STAGE ONE

### Summary——Stage One: **Being**

| | |
|---|---|
| Ego state: | Natural Child |
| Developmental ages: | First week following conception, Birth to 6 months, 13 years |
| | Major recycling begins at 26, 39, 52, 65, 78, 91, etc. |
| Activity: | Needs and feelings |
| Functional metaphor: | Generator |
| Psychoanalytic equivalent: | Early oral |
| Needs: | Feeding and stroking, immediate response to crying signal |
| Developmental focus: | Being rather than doing; building or renewing being touched and having intimate physical contact gathering strength (often by asking others to take over for awhile) taking in being nourished. |
| Key concepts: | Adequacy, supply, using anger to cover fear, basic existential position, dependency, helplessness |
| Chakra: | Root |
| Part of the brain activated: | Medulla and cord |
| Common body symptoms: | Disturbances in the sustaining systems (those without which life cannot continue): immu- |

nologic (susceptibility to infections): digesting (inability to digest foods, ulcers, inflammations); eliminative (constipation, diarrhea); circulatory (impaired circulation, high or low blood pressure); respiratory (wheezing, lowered lung capacity, pneumonia, bronchitis); nervous irritability (hypo— or hyper—reflexes, numbness); blocked genital feelings

| | |
|---|---|
| Problem—solving procedure: | Peek—A—Boo |
| Games and Positions: | NIGYSOB (Now I got you, you S.O.B.), obesity, bag—o—bones, addict, indigent, chain smoker |
| Mechanism: | Denial |
| Injunctions: | Don't be, don't feel, don't have needs |
| Messages in support of *Being* | It's okay for you to be here, to be fed, touched and taken care of. |
| | You have a right to be here. |
| | Your needs are okay with me. |
| | I'm glad you're a (boy/girl). |
| | I like to hold you, to be near you, to touch you. |
| | You don't have to hurry; you can take your time. |

# STAGE ONE

## Activities for Stage One

1. I know when I need to be taken care of for a while because I:

_____am tired                   _____do more and more tasks

_____am irritable               _____eat

_____am depressed               _____starve

_____am nervous                 _____think a lot

_____need more sleep            _____have trouble sleeping

Other: _____

2. When I imagine myself in my life now being taken care of exactly as I want and need, the following scene comes to mind:

_____

_____

_____

3. When I picture the baby I once was and who remains an active, vital part of my life, I feel:

_____scared      _____sad       _____happy      _____joyous

_____depressed   _____enraged   _____panicked

Other: _____

4. What the baby I once was needs to know and hear right now is:

_____

_____

_____

## The Cycle of Life

I will give and receive the messages in support of *Being* to myself and others in the following ways:

_____

_____

_____

# STAGE TWO

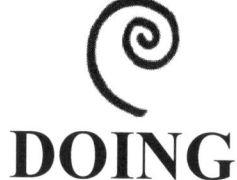

## ◎
# DOING

## The World of Senses and Action

*(Six Months to Eighteen Months)*

*Don't tame the Wild God.*

Chogyam Trungpa

As adults in the exploratory stage, we use our senses to take in information and to learn. We feed ourselves new information about the world via our sight, sound, smell, touch, taste, and kinesthesia, or ability to sense movement. In so doing, we develop our intuition. Our relationships with others are still very much in the joining—with style characteristic of the Being stage, but now we add parallel play. We like to be around others who are also playing and exploring, but we are not yet interested in playing with them other than in an exploratory way. Fulfilling needs of the exploratory stage in this way constructs the necessary links between our dependency—relating of the previous stage and our ability to establish a new level of independence in the next stage.

When we complete unfinished emotional business from the ages of around six to eighteen months, we actively finish building experiences that bridge the gap between our dependency with parents and doing things on our own. We still borrow the functions of thinking and doing as we did in the Being stage. However, as babies we begin to initiate transactions by means other than crying. We can do this because our bodies are developed well enough to sit up and, later, to pick up objects and perceive and crawl towards sources of stimulation. We develop and integrate our senses as we scan our environment much like a radar screen. We are in search of sources of stimulation——sights, sounds, smells, touches, tastes and movement. We use our voluntary nervous system and our skeletal muscles and in so doing, we are activating the neurological connections in the area of our brain called the pons. The pons is a part of our central nervous system that helps regulate our breathing and transmits sensory information between our cerebellum (which helps integrate and coordinate sensory perception and motor output) and cerebrum (which coordinates communication, including language, movement, smell and memory).

This new need to explore the environment in search of sensory experience is a developing capacity that in Transactional Analysis is called the Little Professor. It stretches out from the earlier dependency of the Natural Child like a sprout from a new leaf.

But just as a new leaf withers when it does not receive enough energy to supply it, these new aptitudes wither in people who have to sacrifice their Natural Child Being needs in order to explore. For a baby of this age, not being able to explore is like being asked to starve. If we are required to inhibit our behavior in a certain area ("Don't touch that vase!" "No, no, leave that alone!") we may choose to inhibit all behavior. Since we are too young to limit behavior selectively, we may decide to become passive. The net effect is to undercut our budding motivation.

## Stage Two

Having made this choice of passivity in childhood, we may experience little or no interest in doing things (especially new things) as adults. Our adult behavior is ritualized, listless and lifeless. We have replaced fascination with depression. Or we may have discovered that in our original exploratory experiences we decided that the only way to get attention was to escalate activity. Consequently, we engage in certain behaviors as varied as human imagination. Instead of devoting ourselves to creating the affection and safe exploration that are needed to feed and satisfy our curiosity, we devote ourselves to becoming a "star," or perhaps to excelling at intellectual pursuits in order to get needs met. We may act stupid or sick to win protection and strokes. Some of us may even act constantly happy, or always tough, or fragile. Some of us may decide to be always doing something. In our adult lives, we are all stuck with our "trick," believing it is the only way to get our needs met. If our trick is to do intellectual magic acts, we become more and more heady until we finally drive ourselves to collapse. This set—up is particularly insidious because many of us have become so expert at our trick that our escalation looks like a flash of brilliance or a good feeling, while inside we are feeling more and more pain.

What we need to do is take in through our senses the energy and stimulation that is essential to the development of our physical body and of our voluntary nervous system. When we are deprived of this energy, or are only allowed to explore it when we do tricks, we find that we have behavioral, perceptual and motivational problems. They range from the silly——"I can't hear with my glasses off!"——to the serious, such as sight, hearing and speech difficulties.

The effects of unmet exploratory needs show up in adult behavior as gawkiness, awkwardness or a spastic quality to movements. Blocks in doing things seem to produce physical stress reactions, as if adrenal glands were stuck producing vast amounts of adrenalin. Physically and psychologically we seem "stuck" in one of the self—preservation reactions: fight, flight or freeze.[22] Then we may either heighten our intuition, to sense any possible danger, or we may dull it so as not to be aware of threats.

In some of us a stroke hunger from the previous six months coupled with a stress reaction from this stage results in a hyper—vigilant immune system that responds to everything as an allergen, thus contributing to the symptoms of asthma.

Solving problems from this stage always seems easier than identifying them. We need to have protective, affectionate caring that also supports our need to explore in a sensory way. This is not to imply that we should be indulged with no limits——quite the contrary. If we are exploring and come to a dangerous situation, we need to be supported in finding two "Yesses" instead of only a "No." This is the same kind of creating of options that toddlers need: "You can't bite the lamp cord. Here's a cracker or your teething ring." Once it is safe to follow our noses, we heal physical difficulties easily. If we no longer have to inhibit all behavior, we easily become spontaneous, creative

## STAGE TWO

and motivated. We may report that if we no longer have to pull energy in through our eyes alone, our vision improves.

We can set up experiences where it is okay for us to explore in this way where there is no requirement for us to behave in any one way. We can do what we want to do to feed our senses, including nothing, and we will still be able to maintain the emotionally sustaining relationships we need. We discover that we do not have to sacrifice connection for growth. As grownups, we can now learn that we can always find safe options ("Yesses") instead of repeating dangers or inhibitions ("No, no, no!")[17]

THE CYCLE OF LIFE

**Summary—Stage Two: <u>Doing</u>**

| | |
|---|---|
| Ego state: | Little Professor |
| Developmental ages: | Second and third week in utero, 6 to 18 months, 13 ½ |
| | Major recycling begins at 26 1/2, 39 1/2, 52 1/2, 65 1/2, 78 1/2, 91 1/2, etc |
| Activity: | Behavior |
| Functional metaphor: | Radar |
| Psychoanalytic equivalent: | Oral exploratory |
| Needs: | Exploring and doing things, two for every "No" |
| Developmental focus: | To explore the environment without having to think about it; develop sensory awareness by doing; tasting, touching, smelling, feeling, hearing and seeing what the world is about; feeling the earth, finding footing, getting in touch with the ground; seeking a variety of stimulation; being free to move out into the world and to follow our own urges. |
| Key concepts: | Initiating, motivation, curiosity, creativity, intuition, motion, exploring, options, grounding, using fear to cover anger |
| Chakra: | Hara |
| Part of brain activated: | Pons |

## STAGE TWO

| | |
|---|---|
| Common body symptoms: | Adrenal stress reaction activated with behavior; being stuck in flight, fight or freeze response; sensorimotor impairments (hypo— or hyperactivity); visual/auditory problems; asthma; migraine |
| Problem—solving procedure: | You'll never get away |
| Games and positions: | Do me something, cavalier, sweetheart, me too, harried, asthma, gee you're wonderful, greenhouse |
| Mechanism: | Projection |
| Injunctions: | Don't bother (me); don't initiate, don't do things; don't be curious, real, intuitive |
| Messages in support of *Doing*: | It's okay for you to move out in the world, to feed your senses and be taken care of.<br>It's okay for you to explore and experiment.<br>You can do things and get support at the same time.<br>It's okay for you to initiate.<br>You can be curious and intuitive.<br>You can get attention for the way you really feel. |

# The Cycle of Life

**Activities for Stage Two**

1. I know when I need to explore the possibilities of my life or my environment because:

\_\_\_\_I am restless          \_\_\_\_my production goes way down

\_\_\_\_I am bored           \_\_\_\_my motivation diminishes

\_\_\_\_my concentration is short   \_\_\_\_I need to move, see, and hear new places, people and things

\_\_\_\_my attention wanders    \_\_\_\_thinking about what to do doesn't work

2. When I imagine myself in my life now having the freedom, safety and affection I need to explore exactly as I want and need, the following scene comes to mind:

_____

_____

_____

3. When I picture the toddler I once was who is still an active, vital part of my life, I feel:

\_\_\_\_scared     \_\_\_\_sad       \_\_\_\_happy      \_\_\_\_joyous

\_\_\_\_depressed  \_\_\_\_enraged   \_\_\_\_panicked

Other_____

## Stage Two

4. What that toddler I once was needs to know and hear right now is:

_____

_____

_____


5. I will give and receive new messages about *Doing* to myself in the following ways:

_____

_____

_____

# STAGE THREE

## THINKING

### The Conceptual Realm

*(Eighteen Months to Three Years)*

*No, I won't, and you can't make me.*

Anonymous

When we enter Stage Three, we need to carry out the same growth tasks as do children who are between the ages of about eighteen months to three years. We often report feeling "stuck" and confused. When questioned about our experience, we frequently answer, "I don't know." We report feeling extremely uncomfortable, often tired and "muddy." Attempts by others to interpret this turn of events never work out. In fact, when others think for us, our emotional issues intensify and we become more stuck. Soon everyone is puzzled and more than a few are angry. It looks like a terminal case of resistance.

Actually, we are starting to relate to others in the healthy, contrary, oppositional ways that are characteristic of this stage. We are pushing and testing others, crossing up the "joining with" ways of relating we typically used to the first two stages. We push and challenge others to find their limits, and in so doing, find our own.

Although we don't give others any direct answers during the time we are locked into that experience, we are starting an important emotional development. We are beginning the process of "learning to think." We are gaining the ability to use our own "computer." The long pauses which may puzzle or even anger others, and which they often interpret as resistance, are indications that we are placing our attention internally, to put some order into the sea of sensory experiences we amassed while exploring. We are developing the ability to "remember" at will, thus gaining the capacity to make connections between two or more sensory events. While others are waiting, we are integrating.

We are also establishing our own personal answers to questions such as: "Is it OK for me to be separate?" "Can I become an individual in my own right and still be connected?" "Can I think for myself?" "Do I have to take care of other people by thinking for them, or by deciding not to think?" "What are others' limits?" and "What are my own limits?" We resolve these questions in the healthiest way when we decide to use our capacity to think to solve problems. Those of us who had information withheld from us at this age may feel that our capacity to think and know has been discounted, that is, not taken into account. Our thinking was undercut because, without certain information, we could not adequately assess our needs and feelings. It is hard to prepare for the stimulation of a grocery store, or other such specific destination, when we don't know where we are going until we get there.

We may feel there is a conspiracy afoot to keep us uninformed. As grownups, we may become angry and controlling, stubbornly maintaining a position even if we have made up our minds arbitrarily. This behavior may be evidence of a belief that dependency is not safe. Alternatively, we may appear little and helpless, taking hours to make up our minds only to reverse our decisions, preferring to control situations in that way. It is as if we would rather die than think for ourselves. Such behavior often indicates a belief that independence is not safe.

When we push others for the information we need, they may respond by attempting to control the situation for us. Our pushing can then lead to feeling outright rage. If we try a thought—out approach, asking questions, others may become enraged with *us,* reversing the positions of parent and child in the dependency relationship so that the one who needs parental care becomes the one who takes care of the parents by thinking for them. All of these strategies interfere with our efforts to wire our midbrain (which plays a significant role in motivation) and establish our new ego state, the Adult computer. Leaving these tasks incomplete, we may develop messy, or very tidy, habits. We fend off any external order with a stubborn "I won't," usually cleverly masked behind heightened, or diminished, consciousness and behavior——acting smart or stupid.

We need enough time, enough space, enough strokes, enough information and a loving attitude from others while we learn to think. And we need to do this according to our own motivation rather than someone else's.

The effects of not getting enough time, information and stroking are expressed in our bodies. We have a tightness and stiffness at the base of our necks. Our necks are locked, in an attempt to block more sensory experiences until we have properly integrated the ones already inside. Some of us are oozing energy, while others are "not very together." We may have little energy available except in tight, precise sequences. Attempts to control energy in this way can lead to weight problems. We become overweight or underweight. We eat too much or too little. We have constipation or diarrhea.

Solving problems stemming from this period of our life means getting enough time, information and strokes to maintain the process of integration. We need to experience our own motivation to think, to conceptualize, to find out what we can and cannot control in each situation, and to decide on behavior accordingly. We need to feel safe enough to think about *all* experiences in order to integrate them so that we do not have to sacrifice this need in order to get strokes. Protection at this stage helps us keep sensory input at a level we can handle. It is through this process that we successfully resolve the questions we have raised in this stage. We decide it's okay to be separate, it's okay to have our own limits, and we decide to think to solve problems.

STAGE THREE

**Summary——Stage Three: <u>Thinking</u>**

| | |
|---|---|
| Ego State: | Adult |
| Developmental ages: | Fourth through sixth week in utero |
| | 18 months to 3 years |
| | 14 |
| | Major recycling begins at 28 1/2, 41 1/2, 54 1/2, 67 1/2, 80 1/2, 93 1/2 etc. |
| Activity: | Thinking |
| Functional metaphor: | Computer |
| Psychoanalytic equivalent: | Anal |
| Needs: | Time and information, reasons, limits, affection |
| Developmental focus: | To find out our importance in relation to others, develop concepts, take in information and learn to think, find our limits and those of the world, make connections between sensory events, express negativity and ambivalence, push against others; have what's mine apart from yours, exert our opinion, test reality |
| Key concepts: | Separateness, contrariness, compliance or rebellion, controlling issues, shame, pushing, thinking, resistance, integrating, messiness and tidiness |
| Chakra: | Solar plexus |
| Part of brain activated: | Midbrain |

## The Cycle of Life

| | |
|---|---|
| Common body symptoms: | Uncontrollable discharges of energy, seizures, constipation, stiff neck, central and autonomic nervous systems not together |
| Problem-solving procedure: | Try and make me |
| Games and positions: | Schlemiel, stupid, goody two—shoes, balance sheet, look what you made me do, sunny—side up, tell me this, I'll show them |
| Mechanism: | Discounting |
| Injunctions: | Don't think, don't have needs separate from me, everything is okay with me (because I can't be separate or have boundaries of my own, or my own position) |
| Messages in support of *Thinking:* | It's okay for you to push and test to find limits, to say "No" and become separate from me.<br>You can think for yourself; you don't have to take care of other people by thinking for them.<br>You can be sure about what you need.<br>You can think about your feelings and feel about your thinking.<br>You can let people know when you feel angry.<br>I'm glad you're growing up! |

## Stage Three

**Activities for Thinking**

1. I know when I need to develop and use my capacity to think because I:

\_\_\_\_\_push against others        \_\_\_\_\_want my own position
\_\_\_\_\_oppose what's going on    \_\_\_\_\_become preoccupied with "mine and yours" instead of "ours"
\_\_\_\_\_feel stubborn                    \_\_\_\_\_act rebellious or compliant
\_\_\_\_\_want to say "No" or "I won't"

2. When I imagine myself in my life now having the freedom, safety and affection I need to think for myself, the following scene comes to mind:

_____
_____
_____

3. When I picture the two—year—old I once was who is still an active, vital part of my life I feel:

\_\_\_\_\_scared        \_\_\_\_\_sad        \_\_\_\_\_happy        \_\_\_\_\_joyous
\_\_\_\_\_depressed   \_\_\_\_\_enraged   \_\_\_\_\_panicked
Other_____

4. What the two—year old I once was needs to know and hear right now is:

_____
_____
_____

## THE CYCLE OF LIFE

5. I will give and receive message in support of *Thinking* to myself and others in the following ways:

_____

_____

_____

# STAGE FOUR

# IDENTITY

## Our Ever—Evolving Self

*(Three To Six Years)*

*Always remember that you are absolutely unique.*

*Just like everyone else.*

Margaret Mead

We have now achieved a landmark in our development. We have passed through the first three stages, in which we have answered for ourselves some questions basic to our ability to survive and thrive: "Is it okay for me to be here?" (Stage One), "Is it okay for me to explore and do things?" (Stage Two), and "Is it okay for me to be separate, to think for myself?" (Stage Three). This milestone now poses a new set of questions. Since we exist, can do things, and are separate people, then who are we, and who are all these other people? These are the fundamental questions of our journey through this identity stage.

These inquiries are directly related to the birth and development of a new capacity and part of our personality——the Parent in the Child, or SuperNatural Child. In its negative manifestations, it has also been called the electrode, the witch mother or the troll father.

As we attempt to answer these existential queries, we develop the initial cortex of our brain. Neurologically, we are wiring our nerve cells together so they fire together, then making neuropeptides that send this information throughout our bodies. As our cells receive this information, they change according to the message. The way we wire these things together constitutes our identity.

The capacities we give birth to at this age work like a transformer capable of changing energy from one form to another. We can turn caring into hurting, joy into sorrow, anger into fear, or terror into rage. The fact that we may feel that we do not possess this power is an illusion. We are all powerful, creative beings.

When our developmental process is fixated in unfinished emotional business stemming from the ages of around three to six years old, we often look like we are going crazy or are possessed by the devil. Some of us seem to have an evil quality about us; others act sinister, frightening or powerful. Some of us look weak, like we are going to fall apart at any moment.

One of the first things we notice about ourselves and others is that we are either male or female. We therefore pay close attention to how persons of our own gender or of the opposite gender act. The conclusions we reach at this young age, even if buried in our unconscious, can predetermine the choices we feel are open to us, which become closed for the rest of our adult lives unless we update them.

In this stage we may seem bent on getting our friends to fight with each other. We often report waking with fright from a nightmare. We are actively involved in magical acts——thinking certain thoughts in order to produce certain effects. We report feeling that we have caused events to happen no matter how unrelated to our actions those events seem to other people.

## Stage Four

Transactions initiated towards us are not likely to be taken "straight." We may respond to a caring remark with hurt, or to a happy story with pain and sorrow. For this reason it does not seem possible to talk with us about what is going on until after it has taken place. Meanwhile others hold on to their faith that "We know what we need to do." They assume that somehow we must be doing what we need to do, and that somewhere inside us we know how to respond.

This unlikely process is the one by which we throw off the effect of all the illusions we internalize about who we really are. Our entire collection of illusions about ourselves and others seems to be contained in this ego state, much like a library filled with books. In order to "clean out the shelves" we direct energy through, or "energize," each illusion or image in order to be done with it. We pull the old skeletons out of the closet and try them on like costumes.

The process is more difficult to complete if those around us are "taken in" or caught up in the illusion, reinforcing and validating it as if it were our real selves, rather than a costume. We need to hear that we can act like an ogre and even succeed in frightening people without being basically or intrinsically an ogre.

The more "skeletons" we drag out of the closet, try on and discard, the more we can function in this ego state. The label "SuperNatural Child" is used because this part of us is the channel through which we get in touch with other—than—the—known forces of nature. How we set our channels is called our "script decision."[24] Getting rid of the "skeletons," we open the channel to knowledge of other planes of consciousness. The more open we become, the more we can use our greater intuitive power.

There are guidelines to aid the process. The first and most important guideline is that nobody can do it for us. No matter how strong others' urge to help, to point a better way, ultimately we must each discover for ourselves through our own experiences what is valid for us.

Second, outward appearances notwithstanding, is this: "Everybody is Buddha." In other words, every one of us is innately okay and powerful. Some of us are simply more convincing actors than others.

Third is that people at every age, but especially at this one, are best served by compassionate and total honesty from others. We need straight reactions to events. This means we all must shed as rapidly as possible our illusions about what we are "supposed to be like," or how we are "supposed to react," or about what is "normal" and what is not. We can even joke about how we don't look or act or feel like the "Average Human Being" kept locked in a vault in the Bureau of Standards in Washington, D.C.

While working through problems from this ego state, we report feeling many changes in our physical energy. As we gradually let go of former controls on our aliveness, our consciousness seems to float on a sea of stormy vitality. As we continue our inquiries about who we are and who these other people are, we find balance within ourselves, and in so doing, calm the storm.

## Stage Four

Meanwhile, we are quite susceptible to various illnesses, especially infections and accidents. For that reason it is especially important not to induce stress in relationships by making demands for change, but to offer and receive a lot of physical stroking while the adjustments make themselves.

Sometimes we may feel pain over our heart and in our chest muscles. As we gradually complete answers to who we are and who these other people are, the "electrode activity" begins to settle down and we feel our chest open up. Behaviorally, we are becoming free to love, to care and to "have a heart."

THE CYCLE OF LIFE

## Summary—Stage Four: **Identity**

| | |
|---|---|
| Ego state: | SuperNatural Child |
| Developmental ages: | Seventh through eleventh week in utero, 3 to 6 years, 15 |
| | Major recycling begins at 29, 42, 55, 68, 81, 93, etc. |
| Activity: | Transforming energy |
| Functional metaphor: | Transformer |
| Psychoanalytic equivalent: | Genital |
| Needs: | Adequate external supply lines maintained while testing power |
| Developmental focus: | To find out "Who am I?," create an identity, discover what being male or female means, test definitions of reality through consequences, exert power to affect relationships, separate fantasy from reality, develop the ability to organize and change our internal reality. |
| Key concepts: | Magic, potency/impotency, power, caring/hurting, genital orientation, going crazy/going sane, setting up fights, transformer, electrode, channel |
| Chakra: | Heart |
| Part of brain activated: | Initial cortex |

## Stage Four

| | |
|---|---|
| Common body symptoms: | Circulatory problems, chest pain, palpitations, muscular binding in chest, raised or lowered basal metabolic rate |
| Problem—solving procedure: | Let's pretend |
| Games and positions: | Mine's bigger than yours: let's you and him fight; uproar Rapo; cops and robbers buzz off, buster; let's pull a fast one on Joey; I'm only trying to help |
| Mechanism: | Conversion (repressing an emotion that manifests in a hysterical symptom) |
| Injunctions: | Eat your heart out, don't be sane, don't be powerful, don't be loving, watch out! |
| Messages in support of *Identity*: | It's okay for you to have your own view of the world, to be who you are and to test your power.<br><br>You can be powerful and still have needs.<br><br>You don't have to act scary, sick, sad or mad to get taken care of.<br><br>It's okay for you to explore who you are. It's important for you to find out what you are about. |

## The Cycle of Life

It's okay to imagine things without being afraid you will make them come true.

It's okay for you to find out the consequences of your own behavior.

## STAGE FOUR

**Activities for Stage Four**

1. I know when I need to develop my identity further because I:

   _____ am fascinated with differences  _____ focus on how much I can affect others

   _____ have frequent scary dreams

   _____ experiment with different images of myself

   _____ deal with who I am, who others think I am, who I thought I was and who I can become

2. When I imagine myself in my life now having the freedom, safety and affection I need to explore who I am, the following scene comes to mind:

   _____

   _____

   _____

3. When I picture the preschooler I once was who is still an active, vital part of my life, I feel:

   _____ scared      _____ sad       _____ happy      _____ joyous

   _____ depressed   _____ enraged   _____ panicked

   Other: _____

   _____

   _____

## The Cycle of Life

4. What the preschooler I once was needs to know and hear right now is:
_____
_____
_____

5. I will give and receive messages in support of *Identity* to myself and others in the following ways:
_____
_____
_____

# STAGE FIVE

# SKILLFULNESS

## The "How—To's" of Our Lives

### (Six to Twelve Years)

*An ounce of practice is worth more than tons of preaching.*

Mohandas Gandhi

Having come to our identity conclusions in Stage Four, we are now ready to develop the personal skills we need to get along in the world based on that identity. This gives rise to numerous questions in need of answers: "How am I to act as a member of my gender and culture?" "What behaviors are OK or not OK?" "What do I value?" "How do I deal with those who are older/younger/the same age, my gender/the opposite gender?" "How shall I spend my time?" "What do I need to learn?" and "How do I learn?"

In the initial phase of this stage, we may appear to be reverting to two—year—old behavior. Once more we relate to others in an oppositional or contrary way. We may seem emotionally sullen, sulky, and diffident. Internally, we feel stuck and confused again. Yet others' attempts to help us get unstuck are useless——nothing works, again!

As we begin to put words to these events, we can see that nothing others can offer will work because we are getting ready to have our *own* way of doing things, our own Parent ego state. Our "stuckness" says, "I am going to do it *my* way this time, or not at all!" Gradually our resistance and contrariness bloom into arguing with others.

While this may appear to be aimed at the person we are arguing with, it actually is born of the desire to bring out others' ways of doing things, or others' values, so that we can defend against them long enough to edit them and create a structure that is uniquely our own.

However, many of us were unable to argue and hassle with our parents or other important authorities during our first pass through this stage at ages six through twelve. A variety of reasons for this may be true. For example, a parent may have been absent emotionally or physically, or our arguing was overpowered by an abusive parent, or our parent caved in, unable to stand up to our hassling. Whatever the reason, in our adult life, without even thinking about it, we assume it is dangerous to let anyone know that we want to have our own way of doing things. To complete the developmental tasks of this stage and develop our own internal authority, we need to release ourselves from this inner emotional logjam.

Those of us who took on others' ways instead of creating our own were set up to suffer in doing things because no one else's way exactly fits our nature. We may feel rigid, stiff and inflexible in our bodies and our lifestyles. We may spend a lot of energy trying to please others, or to get others to please us. We may experience life as one horrendous experiment being conducted upon us by some mad scientist.

If we can only figure out the formula, we'll be able to run through the maze to our great experimental reward. We get more exhausted than depressed because we have engaged in frantic spurts of activity searching for the "key" or the "secret." Many of us in our adult lives have joined group after group of people who claim to know "the secret." Frequently this has cost us our health and, more often than not, our wealth.

We need to find out we can disagree with others' ways with no risk to their stability or our own well—being. That frees us to begin putting together our own ways of doing things. For this purpose we need many experiences of doing things our own way, and we need to argue and hassle with others about their ways. This developmental task helps reorganize the part of our brain called the early cortex.

The idea that it might be *fun* to do things——or even that it is *possible* to learn to do things, let alone have fun in the process——is inconceivable. If learning has always been full of pain, we believe there are too many trials and tribulations along its road. Life is serious after all, we say to ourselves, not something to play around with or make light of. "Toe the line!" "Knuckle under!" "Concentrate!" and "Push!" are some of the the messages we may hear. But our inner child has not been completely blinded to other possibilities. After all, there really *are* a few competent souls out there to model for us.

To learn how to do things our own way we need to take in new ways of doing things — newParent structures to replace the old, painful ones. In letting go of old ways of doing things, based on somebody else's way, we begin to find our own way, based on our own needs. Then our Parent ego state belongs to us, not to some external authority. We need to design it to serve our own internal Child. The machine must be built to serve the person, not vice—versa. This simple fact may be a revelation: we have built part of our personality upside down!

Next, we will need to replace other structures. We find that looking at anything in terms of good and bad, or right or wrong, or making mistakes, is not problem solving at all. We simply have to deal with what works.

Now we are freed to get our personal technology together. How are we going to get our needs met? We need to know how to be angry with a friend, or with a stranger, and resolve it, and how to express fear in such a way as to get reassurance. Then there is the big issue of stroke supply. How can we get strokes? When is it okay, and when not okay? Can boys stroke girls, can women stroke men, can people of the same sex stroke each other, and under what circumstances? We especially love having a same—sex best friend or buddy while we explore the cultural rules for our gender. We cannot learn what being male is all about from females; likewise women can't learn about being female from men. We need these relationships with peers to provide a variety of points of view while we answer questions such as:

What will increase the odds of getting the responses we want in our relationships with others?

How can two people have needs and feelings at the same time, and both get their needs met?

And money:

Is it all right to have money, or not to have money?

How much money should we have?

## STAGE FIVE

What are the right ways to get, keep and spend it?

What ways of doing things do others find oppressive?

What about caring: Can we care for each other without having to sell each others' souls in the process?

How do we relate to power?

Is it all right to have power over other people?

We discover what will work for us by what we disagree with. Each person's behavior, tic or grimace becomes open to scrutiny. We want enough time now to think about things carefully before we make ideas our own.

The process of letting go of an old structure and taking in a new one requires us to be active. We need to try out the new way, reconsider it, alter it a bit, consult about it, and then repeat it many more times until it becomes an automatic part of us.

Frequently we need to do things to let go of a reservoir of psychic energy that had been stopped up by having to run against someone else's gates. Physical activity often opens blocks, especially the painful place between the shoulder blades where we have been allowing the "monkey on our back" to ride. Our posture then improves.

Many of us discover that because we were unable to argue with people of the opposite sex, we had unwittingly incorporated the opposite—sex structures into our Parent. Then we feel that something is wrong with us as sexual beings and that we are unlike others of our sex. Our opposite—sex ways make our physical appearances odd, as if trying to look nonchalant while wearing mother's or father's clothes.

## The Cycle of Life

As we build up our own technological wardrobe, we gain more control until finally we are able to energize our full power at will, signaling the birth of the last component of our personality structure: our separate Parent ego state. It is the voice of our own internal authority——confident, powerful and completely our own.

We experience enough protection to give birth to our own Parent when we are able to examine many ways of doing things, when we are able to choose our own way and let others know what it is without any cost to our stroke supply or integrity, and when we are able to continue structuring without having to structure for other people against our will.

STAGE FIVE

## Summary—Chapter Five: <u>**Skillfulness**</u>

Ego state: Parent

Developmental ages: Twelfth through twenty—fourth week in utero
6—12 years, 16
Major recycling begins at 32, 45, 58, 71, 84, 97, etc.

Activity: Structuring, developing skills

Functional metaphor: Regulator

Psychoanalytic
equivalent: Latency

Needs: Experiences in doing things, hassling to incorporate structures

Developmental focus: To experiment with different ways of doing things; develop physical, intellectual, emotional and social skills; argue, hassle and disagree; exclude others' methods until we make our own; learn new morals, manners or values; make mistakes to find out what works

Key concepts: Doing or not doing things, independence, disagreeing, hassling, arguing, suffering around doing things, latent homosexuality, incorporating structures, making not okay, excluding sex role behaviors

Chakra: Throat (communication)

Part of brain activated: Early cortex

| | |
|---|---|
| Common body problems: | Opposite—sex distribution of fatty tissue, muscular binding in chest area |
| Problem—solving procedure: | Dress up |
| Games and positions: | Courtroom, ain't it awful, blemish, PTA, NIGYSOB (Now I got you, you SOB), kick me |
| Mechanism: | Exclusion |
| Injunctions: | Don't think, just do it; don't structure, don't exclude; don't make mistakes |
| Messages in support of *Skillfulness:* | It's okay for you to learn how to do things your own way, to have your own morals and methods.<br><br>You don't have to suffer to get what you need.<br><br>Trust your feelings to guide you.<br><br>You can think before you make that your way.<br><br>It's okay to disagree.<br><br>You can do it your way. |

STAGE FIVE

**Activities for Stage Five**

1. I know when I am developing my ability to structure and become skillful because I:

\_\_\_\_\_argue with others

\_\_\_\_\_defend against advice

\_\_\_\_\_experience a negative attitude

\_\_\_\_\_make others' ways not okay

\_\_\_\_\_become preoccupied with how things work

\_\_\_\_\_question my own and others' morals and values

\_\_\_\_\_defend against advice

\_\_\_\_\_feel stubborn about values

2. When I imagine myself in my life now having the freedom, safety and affection to develop my own ways and skills, the following scene comes to mind:

_____

_____

_____

3. When I picture the six— to twelve—year—old child I once was who is still an active vital part of my life, I feel:

\_\_\_\_\_ scared  \_\_\_\_\_sad  \_\_\_\_\_happy  \_\_\_\_\_joyous

\_\_\_\_\_ depressed  \_\_\_\_\_enraged  \_\_\_\_\_panicked

Other: _____

4. What that child I once was needs to know and hear right now is:

_____

_____

_____

5. I will give and receive new messages about *Skillfulness* to myself and others in the following ways:

_____

_____

_____

_____

_____

# STAGE SIX

# REGENERATION

## Creation and Procreation

*(Thirteen to Nineteen Years)*

> *Character cannot be developed in ease and quiet.*
> *Only through experience of trial and suffering can*
> *the soul be strengthened, ambition inspired, and*
> *success achieved.*
>
> Helen Keller

Having completed Stage Five, we now have built all the components of our personality. Again, this gives rise to a new emotional need: to integrate these component parts into one functioning whole. When we begin this stage, initially we are also integrating the many physical and emotional events of puberty, beginning the changes that will result in our ability to procreate——to give birth to a new generation.

To integrate all these internal parts along with the changes of puberty, we repeat all our previous stages again in rapid succession as we finalize our pass through one full cycle of emotional development. In so doing, we are rewiring and reorganizing the part of our brain called our primitive cortex.

First, like the infants we once were, we again eat all the time; we want to be fed, taken care of, and thought *for*. We have high stroking needs. We are concerned about money as an energy supply, and we spend a lot of time preoccupied with sex. We have an incredibly short attention span and are overcome by waves of energy filled with strange, unfamiliar urges——erotic, exciting and scary. We need to

# The Cycle of Life

have our external supply needs met——we need to be fed and taken care of in a loving way. This recommencement through the stages begins at about age thirteen.

Next we revisit our exploratory time. We want periods of time in which to explore in the pre—conceptual world of our senses; to move, touch, smell, hear, see and taste the world again.

Then (around fourteen years old initially) we may be stubborn, negative, compliant or rebellious, depending on our mood. We may be messy. We say "I forgot..." as the bathtub overflows into the downstairs. We are testing control and establishing a thinking position in the social world.

Next (age fifteen at first) we revisit our identity stage. We become preoccupied with who we are, and who we are in relation to others. We test our power to affect other people and experiment with many images, both positive and negative, about who we are and who we can become.

Then (age sixteen initially) we want to argue and hassle. We try to figure out ways not to do something the way others want us to do it. During this pass through the cycle we are getting ready for a friendly divorce from those upon whom we have depended.

Finally, we want to emerge from our parenting or dependency relationship as separate, complete and whole. We still need the protection of our connections with others, and we definitely still have needs, but we are ready to get these needs met from a larger world. We have assumed responsibility for our own needs, our own feelings, and our own behavior as grown—up people in the world.

Those of us whose scripts say "Don't grow up" may feel that our emerging sexuality is the worst trauma that could possibly befall us. Our behavior telegraphs, "Oh no! The one thing that's never supposed to happen is happening! I'm becoming sexual!"

We try various means to compensate. We may wear loose, sloppy clothing to hide our body outlines, or we may always look prim, proper and tidy. We may be more than willing to be honest in the taking care of others, but not in relating to them sexually. We fear being honest about how we feel because we are ashamed of our sexuality. We expect to lose the stroking and protection we need if we let people know we are experiencing sexual feelings.

Those of us whose scripts say "Hurry up and grow up!" may try to use our emerging sexuality to get our dependency needs met. We are likely to tell sexual jokes, comment on our latest sexual event (fantasy or reality), and act blatantly seductive. We have no time for nurturing. We're looking for some "real action!"

Our sexual encounters are ill—fated because they are angry, grown—up attempts to meet the needs of a frightened, helpless child. We may band together in tight, protective cliques to attempt to force what we need from the world.

When we take the position that "Even adolescent problems can be solved, even those of us old enough to be sexual can get our needs met," we can clarify what those needs really are. We need to share our feelings and gather information about our identity as sexual beings in a sexual world. We need to know how others experience their sexuality, and what they do about it. We must learn how to begin and maintain healthy relationships as sexual beings. We need to learn how to handle the possibilities of pregnancy and venereal disease. And we need to learn how to say no to sexual invitations and still be okay.

STAGE SIX

**Summary—Stage Six: <u>Regeneration</u>**

| | |
|---|---|
| Ego state: | Recycling through previous stages |
| Developmental ages: | Twenty—fifth through thirty—sixth weeks in utero, 13 — 18 years, (This stage contains the "Repeat yourself similarly" instruction to recycle; thus this stage repeats, in addition to the other five, after adolescence.) |
| Activity: | Unifying previous activities |
| Functional metaphor: | Integrator, pre—flight |
| Psychoanalytic equivalent: | Puberty |
| Needs: | Work through previously unsolved problems, sex information |
| Developmental focus: | To integrate sexuality with needs from other stages, grow beyond our parenting (or mentoring) relationship, develop our own personal philosophy, develop as a sexually mature person, revisit each earlier stage and update it if necessary, develop a place among grownups, prepare to succeed in the world as a grownup. |
| Key concepts: | Sexuality, recycling of previous stages, unifying functions, integrating personal identity, using cultural parent, breaking family rule |
| Chakra: | Third eye |
| Part of brain activated: | Primitive cortex |

Common body
symptoms:   Delay in sexual development; involutional depressive reactions, both male and female; acne

Note: The following components of Stage Six, identified in the descriptions of the previous stages, are repeated in Stage Six: Problem—solving procedure, Games and positions, Mechanism, Injunctions, and Messages in support of the Stage.

# STAGE SIX

**Activities for Stage Six**

1. I know I am revisiting my adolescent stage of development when I:

\_\_\_\_\_ feel little and all grown—up at the same time

\_\_\_\_\_ want to be on my own/need to be taken care of

\_\_\_\_\_ experience many different stages in rapid succession

\_\_\_\_\_ am preoccupied with sexuality

\_\_\_\_\_ develop my own personal philosophy

\_\_\_\_\_ experience turbulent physical changes, often including acne

2. When I imagine myself in my life now having the freedom, safety and affection I need to deal with my adolescent needs, the following scene comes to mind:

_____

_____

_____

3. When I picture the adolescent I once was who is still an active, vital part of my life, I feel:

\_\_\_\_\_ scared    \_\_\_\_\_ sad    \_\_\_\_\_ happy    \_\_\_\_\_ joyous

\_\_\_\_\_ depressed    \_\_\_\_\_ enraged    \_\_\_\_\_ panicked

Other: _____

4. What the adolescent I once was needs to know and hear right now is:

_____

_____

_____

5. I will give and receive messages in support of *Regeneration* to myself and others in the following ways:

_____

_____

_____

# STAGE SEVEN

# RECYCLING

## Manifesting the Promise of Life

*(Adulthood)*

*What is an adult?*
*A child blown up by age.*

Simone de Beauvoir

And so at last, having integrated to a greater or lesser extent all the parts of ourselves we have been developing until now, we have arrived at the promised land of adulthood. The apparatus of our bodies and personalities we have been building and organizing has so far all been preparation for our arrival into this magical—sounding condition of being grown up. Now, we're ready to see what it's all about.

Adulthood represents a shift from creating the foundation for our lives to building, layer by layer, upon that foundation. By now we've been through the cycle enough times to have some idea of how to handle its stages and growth tasks. Our first acquaintance with it was in the world of water, between our conception and birth, when our growth energy going through each stage was focused on growing our bodies with all their basic parts and downloading very primitive learning systems from our mothers about how to run those bodies.

We added a second layer of programming as we went through a shorter cycle during our birth transition from the world of water to the world of air. Once born, we added a third layer, built on the other two, as we constructed the foundational experiences and laid down the fundamental programming upon which we would build our grown—up lives. Then during adolescence we integrated all these separate stages along with their encoded primal childhood experiences. We worked to become consolidated, unified so that we could function as an adult in the world of adults.

Some of us may interpret the shift in our progress through life from creating a foundation to building upon it as a signal that we should put away the things of childhood. We believe——in fact want to believe——that we've "arrived," and therefore no longer have any more stages to go through or growth tasks to carry out. However, nothing could be further from the truth, for the repetitions of the cycle and its stages persist throughout adulthood. We continue to undergo a major biological repetition of the stages every thirteen years until we draw our last breath.

In addition, each new relationship, each life event adds a repetition of the cycle on top of the biological one. For example, we may be in Stage Four, *Identity,* in our biological repetition, Stage Three, *Thinking,* in our marriage, Stage Five, *Skills,* in our work life and Stage One, *Being,* as we become parents of a child. All these "whorls upon whorls" add psychological and emotional complexity to our inner lives at the same time that we grapple with the challenges of our outer world. In so doing, we are wiring, organizing and calling forth the skills and abilities of the part of our brain called our sophisticated cortex.

## STAGE SEVEN

A key factor affecting how we manage each cyclic revolution in adulthood is the fact that we construct our grown—up lives on the foundation we have already laid down. As adults we are obliged to rely on the information contained in our extra—genetic learning system, whether or not parts are complete, only partially assembled or missing altogether. This means that as the cycle turns, it can activate foundation—level programming and problems. The weight of our adult lives can crack weakly constructed areas, causing the collapse of what we've attempted to build above it. Each return can also expose "hot spots"——emotionally charged memories in need of healing——that cause surface—level volcanic eruptions and earthquakes.

To avoid these eruptions or to attempt stabilization, we may turn to relationships with others. We may try to keep ourselves in a position of control, of being in charge, of taking care of others. Or we may create relationships with others who will take care of us, who will control situations to make sure we get to stay the child——we get to be the one who is taken care of. These are evidence of the fact that we have moved from writing our life stories to playing them out, stage by stage, in our grown—up lives.

Whether we cooperate, control or simply cope, the cycle continues to unfold, gradually shifting our developmental focus with each repetition. In the beginning phases of adulthood, we use the stages to establish ourselves, to build a life structure, find our place, our people, our social milieu. We coalesce and strengthen our separate self, our ego. In following turns we focus on settling in, with some adjustments made to our life structure. It is a time of manifesting our abilities, talents, and, along with them, our developmental deficits. The rotations of later life involve adjusting to the involution of our reproductive capacities and grappling with our ever—increasing awareness of our own mortality. These can give birth to an active interest in our development as spiritual beings, which in turn provides meaning to our later years. Whereas the stages of childhood focused on the development of our selves in the physical and material world, and the stages of early and mid—adulthood centered on action in world, the later turnings begin our ascent out of the material world and into the life of the spirit.

Whether in the beginning, middle or later phase of adulthood, smooth passage from stage to stage depends on our cooperating with our cyclic growth tasks and cleaning up any unfinished business from our inner lives as we evolve. Tools to aid this process are the subject of Part Three.

## STAGE SEVEN

### Summary—Stage Seven: <u>**Recycling**</u>

| | |
|---|---|
| Ego state: | All |
| Developmental ages: | Biological repetitions every thirteen years; timing of harmonic and trigger repetitions vary. |
| Activity: | Establishing independent self in the adult world, creating a life structure, finding our place, living in and modifying our life structure, coming to terms with our culture, manifesting our abilities, reproducing (symbolically through acts and through having children), adjusting to reproductive involution, life review and beginning ascent into spiritual world. |
| Functional metaphor: | Flying |
| Psychoanalytic equivalent: | Adulthood |
| Needs: | Work with our cyclic repetitions, cooperate with and carry out growth tasks of each stage as they present themselves, greet disturbances in our inner lives as opportunities to heal and grow. |
| Developmental focus: | Explore, discover, establish, live out, and later surrender adult roles; regenerate our species by becoming parents or symbolically through mentoring, contribute to projects, etc.; live and modify our personal philosophy and values. |

# The Cycle of Life

Key concepts: Life structure, life story, recycling of previous stages, unifying functions, integrating personal identity, editing, living and changing cultural values, regeneration

Chakra: Third eye

Part of brain activated: Sophisticated cortex

Note: The following components of Stage Seven vary depending on the part of the cycle being revisited: Body Symptoms, Problem-solving procedure, Games and positions, Mechanism, Injunctions, and Messages in support of the Stage.

STAGE SEVEN

**Activities for Stage Seven**

The following are ways we can assess how we're doing in each stage. We can use these statements to assist us in discerning our development. Use a scale of one to ten with one being lowest functioning and ten being highest. The lower a score on any particular item, the more likely we need to pay closer attention to the inner work we need to carry out in that stage, watching for the possibility that we have some unfinished business to complete.

*Stage One*

I am able to:

_____Create the bonds with others that sustain me

_____Discern and decide for myself when to trust and when not to trust

_____Know what I feel——scared, sad, mad, glad…

_____Be aware of when I am tired or hungry and take care of myself accordingly.

*Stage Two*

I am able to:

_____Find ways to satisfy my curiosity in healthy ways

_____Provide for enough variety in my life to keep myself refreshed

_____Balance sufficient activity with times of adequate rest

_____Maintain my sustaining connections with others while exploring

## The Cycle of Life

*Stage Three*

I am able to:

____ Know where I stop and someone else begins

____ Create and maintain healthy boundaries

____ Recognize others' boundaries and respect them whether or not I like or agree with them

____ Think about myself, my own life, my own problems and think to find solutions

____ Be responsible for my commitments, including my word with other people

*Stage Four*

I am able to:

____ Establish who I am in a group of others without overpowering or alienating others or giving up myself

____ Explore my ability to affect others in positive ways

____ Update my sense of self and who I am rather than being rigid, fixated

____ Move from periods of uncertainty about myself and my role in the social world to become at peace with who I am

____ Accept and deal with the consequences of my own behavior

____ Allow others to accept and learn from the consequences of their own behavior–or not learn, as they choose.

STAGE SEVEN

*Stage Five*

I am able to:

\_\_\_\_\_Periodically update my skills

\_\_\_\_\_Review what I value as I grow older, and reset my priorities

\_\_\_\_\_Exhibit tolerance for others' ways of doing things

\_\_\_\_\_Contribute to society in positive ways

\_\_\_\_\_Disagree with others without blaming or criticizing them

\_\_\_\_\_Recognize and respectfully decline invitations to be used

*Stage Six*

I am able to:

\_\_\_\_\_Adjust to my changing sexual maturity as I grow through early, middle and older adulthood

\_\_\_\_\_Accept increasing responsibility for the contents of my life and make the changes I deem necessary to carry them out

\_\_\_\_\_Express my creativity in ways that are healthy for me and for society

\_\_\_\_\_Find ways to stand up to social injustice that do not harm me or others

\_\_\_\_\_Recognize that the world does not owe me a living, and stand on my own two feet; support myself

\_\_\_\_\_Accept support from others and support others in mutually beneficial exchanges

\_\_\_\_\_Take responsibility for my own health and well—being and make the life adjustments that will maintain them.

\_\_\_\_\_Acknowledge that my own reservoir of personal pain exists and take effective steps to heal it.

# PART THREE

# CREATING SMOOTH PASSAGES

*...do not be afraid to investigate the worst.*
*It only guarantees increase of soul power.*

Clarissa Pinkola Estes

In Part Two, we became familiar with each of the seven stages of our recurring cycle in general. Carrying out the exercises, we began to become aware of our own relationship to each stage.

Part Three addresses how to begin to work with our cycle when we encounter areas in which we are tripping, stumbling, falling, failing to succeed. These may be as simple as neglecting to carry out the tasks of the stage, or they may represent earthquakes or eruptions from the underground levels of our extra—genetic programming. How then do we cope, recover——or even heal? How do we get back on track and turn apparently unconscious self—sabotage into satisfaction and success, becoming more fully who we are in the process? To do so, we must greet these rather unwelcome experiences as invitations. This is the topic addressed in the following pages.

# BEGINNING

*Worldly power means nothing.*
*Only the unsayable, jeweled inner life matters.*

Jelaluddin Rumi

The very fact that our inner process is cyclic means we have opportunities not only to carry out our current growth tasks, but also to heal any past traumas, resolve any internal conflicts, free ourselves from internal pain, release ourselves from any previously imposed limits, and liberate ourselves to pursue our own dreams instead of long—forgotten illusions. This is indeed good news.

Ancient wisdom reminds us that when we try to forget the past we condemn ourselves to repeat it. This is a primary source of our self—sabotage. When we have unfinished emotional business from foundation life experiences——no matter from what stage of the cycle——we build an entire structure around it. This can involve feelings, original pain, negative beliefs, perspectives on life, distorted thinking, blocks and defenses, even neurological circuitry and patterning. Happily, we transform this entire construction as we complete our healing and return to the natural process as the stages of our lives unfold. We can relax into its natural pattern, maximizing our potential for growth, health and satisfaction.

How do we go from intellectually knowing we have some unfinished business from these stages, to successfully dealing with it? The first step often is realizing that we *can*, that it is possible, and that we deserve to do it. The beginning is starting to view ourselves as we really are——unique and powerful beings.

As we begin to focus our attention on what is going on in ourselves, we're likely to encounter different voices in our head, not all of which are in agreement with each other. This is a reflection of how we are made. as neurologist Paul D. MacLean tells us in his work on the triune brain. He observed that we think we have one mind but that actually we have three, one built upon the other. He called these the reptilian brain ("archipallium"), limbic system ("palleomammilian") and neocortex ("neopallium").[25]

We experience the functions of this biological design when we transact with others through our ego states, or states of the self.[20] Classified by psychiatrist Eric Berne, he named three main ego states. As grownups each of us experiences them internally as three primary voices that together form our completed personality structure. These organs of consciousness Berne named Parent, Adult and Child, with typical perspectives as follows:

Parent    (P)    "I should"

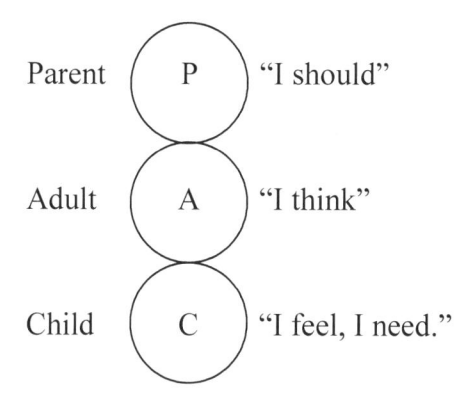

Adult    (A)    "I think"

Child    (C)    "I feel, I need."

These three ego states actually function like three distinct beings within each of us. We hear our Parent say: "I should." It judges and moralizes: "You should do this, you shouldn't do that." Meanwhile, our Adult says "I think." It is able to compute, being our rational self which can figure out practical solutions to problems using "data" from our experiences. Our Child says "I feel, I need," and can dream, wish and even have tantrums. It is the source of our creative energy.

If we feel pulled in several directions about a decision, we are likely to be hearing different instructions from each voice. Our Parent might say, for example, "You should *not* go to the beach today. It's utterly irresponsible!" while our Adult might say, "Today is Sunday. It's warm and sunny. The weather report is consistent with beach weather." Meanwhile our Child is simply saying, "I wanna go. I wanna. I wanna!"

After acknowledging our ability to do so, the second step in discovering what is going on in our inner selves is *hearing* the voices within us and identifying them as Parent, Adult or Child so that we know who is speaking. This involves *listening* to each voice so that we know

"What is the message? Is it healthy? Does it lead to a resolution of the situation, or does it make matters worse? How is it affected by other messages? Is there a balance between them?" If our Child feels weak in the face of a strong Parental "You should!" it is goodbye to the beach for today at least, other options notwithstanding.

## Activities for Beginning

Think of a decision you need to make and use it to complete the following sentences.

1. The voice of our Child ego state talks about feelings, wants and needs. For example:

"I feel... (mad, sad, happy, guilty, scared, delighted, etc.)."

"I want... (a new car, a vacation, a massage, a day in the sunshine, etc.)."

"I need... (a good night's sleep, more exercise, a good breakfast, etc.)."

Now, complete the following sentences:

My Child often feels _____

My Child wants _____

My Child needs _____

2. The voice of our Adult ego state is like a computer that reports thinking. For example, "I think... (that 2 +2 = 4, that the moon is almost full, that there is less traffic after sundown, that it is raining now, etc.)."

Now, complete the following:

My Adult thinks _____

3. The voice of our Parent ego state talks about values and morals. For example, "I should... (finish this project, save my money, pay my taxes, exercise every day, brush my teeth, etc.)."

Now complete the following:

My Parent says I should _____

4. We may experience a conflict in an area of our lives such as following a diet, being on time for appointments, spending money.

Use this exercise as an example:

My Parent says, "I should exercise every day."

My Adult reports these facts: "It is possible to do; other people do it."

"I am a busy person."

"The information about how to do it is available."

My Child says, "I wanna play. I'm tired. Reading this novel is more fun."

Now, complete the following:

5. An area of my life in which I experience a conflict is:
_____
_____

In regard to this conflict:

My Child often feels
_____

My Adult thinks _____

My Parent says I should _____

What I will do is _____

In relating to others, we can also hear these three parts. In so doing we open up a variety of options for relating between their Parent, Adult and Child and our own.

# BEGINNING

6. A conflict I experience in a relationship is about
_____

7. In regard to this conflict

My Child feels _____

My Adult thinks_____

My Parent says I should _____


8. About this conflict, the other person's

Child feels_____

Adult thinks_____

Parent says they should_____

# WISELY MEETING OUR NEED FOR RECOGNITION

*In grown—ups, the symbolic equivalent of the handling of infants is recognition and has survival value.*

Eric Berne

Our progression though life is not only individual, it is also relational. This fact becomes evident as each of us struggles to come to terms with our own unique history, for such historical business is always with *someone* individually or several *someones* collectively. And what others say or do radically aids or detracts from our healing process.

Many of us may have fooled ourselves into believing that life is just one disappointment after another, that there is no light at the end of the tunnel, and that maybe there isn't even a tunnel! On the other hand, we may believe people who say "All you have to do is think positively and brush your teeth every day and everything will turn out all right."

Occasionally, though, we may see something different. We may spend a few hours giggling with a friend, just like kids. Someone may have said something so endearing and funny that we reach over and hugged them. Or perhaps a friend said, "You look wonderful!" Some of us were taught to believe that these messages are too insignificant to make a difference in our lives. It is, however, these very same exchanges that can restore us emotionally and connect us to our high and energetic spaces. Lacking them, we feel unloved and physically depressed. Accepting affectionate, affirming exchanges with others, we no longer keep ourselves down. Such exchanges can feel as if "a physical exchange takes place, as if some substance were passing directly to the cells."[27]

As babies, we needed strokes as much as we needed food. If we hadn't had enough strokes, ultimately we would have died![28] Babies need to be patted and cuddled. Children need to be touched and loved because physical strokes are an essential source of fuel, just as food is a source of energy. Children who get too little stroking become uninterested in their surroundings and withdraw from the world.

We grownups are no different from babies in this respect. We all need a supply of this emotional food to keep our bodies functioning and healthy. We also need stroking. We need to be touched, recognized and gentled. Just as other animals have their grooming rituals, so we have our stroking rules and rituals. Whether we realize it consciously or not, we are often careful not to make any choices that adversely affect our supply of strokes. Our behavior is often determined by what we feel we can afford ——in the supply of and demand for strokes.

We can learn a great deal about how we run our lives, or how our lives run us, by examining our past with the idea of strokes in mind. If we think about it, we can see in which exchanges with others we felt high and energetic, in which ones we felt sad, and how our choices were affected by our stroke supply.

## Wisely Meeting Our Need for Recognition

We can also learn a great deal about our relationships by paying attention to the exchange of strokes. We gravitate to certain relationships and avoid others in large part based on the strokes we can give and receive in them.

We can identify the rules by which we seek or decide to accept strokes. Some of us were taught that we cannot ask for strokes or, even worse, that we should not need them. Children may run into a room, crawl into a lap and ask for a hug, but adults behaving in such a way infringe on social rules and risk being cut off from further stroking.

However, believing that we can't ask for strokes does not change the fact that we need them. When we believe we are only allowed the needs that are "on the menu" for the day, and strokes are not listed, we are in a quandary. Should we change the menu? Or should we go underground instead, indirectly seeking what we need by playing a *game*?

**Activities for Strokes**

My favorite strokes I like to give to myself are:

    1._____
    2._____
    3._____
    4._____
    5._____

The strokes I like to give to others are:

    1._____
    2._____
    3._____
    4._____
    5._____

The strokes I like to receive from others are:

    1._____
    2._____
    3._____
    4._____
    5._____

Strokes I decided never to accept, no matter how badly I may want or need them are:

    1._____
    2._____
    3._____
    4._____
    5._____

# PLAYING IT STRAIGHT

*Games are substitutes for the real living of real intimacy.*

Eric Berne

If we don't ask directly for what we need, and if we don't want to starve, we can "go a—fishin'." We spend our psychic energy playing games in an attempt to get our needs met indirectly.[29] If we are clever and dedicated, we can manipulate the situation so that what we are fishing for takes the bait and we can feel as if we have won. However, playing games ultimately leads to deprivation, because it requires more energy than it returns. It takes more energy to reach a goal by an indirect route than by a direct one. In other words, it takes more energy to be passive about a problem than to be active about it.

When we deplete or dam up our reserves of energy we are, in effect, starving ourselves. Our energy is either gone or unavailable, and we feel even needier. We may decide to play another harder game to "up the ante," hoping for a better return in a maneuver called "escalation."

Escalation is the process by which we wall off or drain psychic energy in an attempt to render it inactive. Four types of behavior signal escalation. Each can follow the other in a step—like progression unless we reverse the process.

## The Four Passive Behaviors Signaling Escalation[30]

1. Doing nothing (relevant to a need or problem we have)
2. Over—adapting (doing what someone else's Parent says to do, instead of doing what we need to do)
3. Becoming agitated (emotionally disturbed, worked up)
4. Becoming incapacitated or violent (imploding, that is, going crazy; or exploding, for example, hitting someone)

If we fail to ask for what we need directly, we can choose our kind of escalation from the many varieties of games. Our game choice in a particular situation is often determined by how many strokes we can get. Usually the larger the potential stroke yield, the more attractive the game. However, since our position is that we cannot get what we need, we set up the situation so that we get only what we think is available—— negative strokes. These are some examples:

- We run ourselves down whenever someone compliments us.
- We pick a fight for no apparent reason.
- We act increasingly incompetent until someone reacts negatively to us.
- We fuss about others' actions until we feel justified in raging about their incompetence.

Many of us go through our lives asking for and getting negative strokes. We become more and more unhappy and unable to change things. We expect bad things to happen to us, and we act out the same scenes again and again with the same results. This kind of "set" behavior is often the result of a problem started long ago in our childhood, when negative strokes were the only kind of recognition we could safely receive. The "set" or pattern has become part of our *script*.

Additionally, playing games limits our relationship options to only those roles involved in games, namely Persecutor, Rescuer and Victim. When we recognize these roles, we start to regain our power to transcend them. Otherwise we spend our relationships in this Drama Triangle, changing between the confines of these three roles.[31]

## Activities for Games

Feeling bad is an indication that we may be involved in a game.

The bad feelings I often have are:

1._____

2._____

3._____

4._____

For each feeling listed above, write below the limiting belief that led to this feeling. For example:

**Feeling**         **Belief**

a. boredom          a. I can't get the pleasurable stimulation I need.
b. sadness          b. Life is one loss after another.
c  guilt            c. If I make my own choices, I will suffer the consequences.

_____

_____

_____

Now, complete the following:

| Feeling | Belief |
|---------|--------|
| 1.      | 1.     |
| 2.      | 2.     |
| 3.      | 3.     |
| 4.      | 4.     |

Now, consider how much longer you want to continue reinforcing limiting beliefs instead of getting what you need. For each belief listed above, write down the kind of reinforcement you really need and want, as in the following example:

| **Limiting Belief** | **What I Need to Know** |
|---------------------|-------------------------|
| a. I can't get the pleasurable stimulation I need. | a. I can get all the protection and support I need to explore my world safely. |
| b. My life is one loss after another. | b. People care about me and will stick around; I can rely on others to be there for me. |
| c. If I make my own choices I will suffer the consequences. | c. The more I actively and freely make my own choices, the more I benefit myself and those around me. |

# The Cycle of Life

Next, complete the following:

| **Limiting Belief** | **What I Need to Know** |
|---|---|
| 1. _____ | 1. _____ |
| 2. _____ | 2. _____ |
| 3. _____ | 3. _____ |
| 4. _____ | 4. _____ |

When we find ourselves switching roles on the Drama Triangle, instead of merely reversing roles we have the option of stepping off from any of the three positions of Victim, Persecutor or Rescuer. The following are guides to doing so:

We know we're in the Victim role when we think things like "Poor me," "Why does this always happen to me?" "There's nothing I can do about it." "It's their fault," etc.

**From this Victim role**, we can own our feelings and needs.

State: I want_____

I need_____

I feel_____

We know we're in the Persecutor role when we think things such as "They are… (bad, evil, wicked)," "They deserve to be punished," "I'll get them," "They'll be sorry," etc.

**From the Persecutor role**, we can create a clear structure to get to our goal. We can make a set of instructions in the same way we would give directions to go from one place to another:

"First do this _____

Then do this _____

Then this" _____

We know we're in the Rescuer role when we think things like "You can't help it," "Let me do that for you" (even though you can and should do it for yourself), "There, there, it's not your fault" (even though it is), etc.

**From the Rescuer role**, we can provide clear nurturing for ourselves internally or for others in relationships. For example, we can use the ultimate nurturing message, or a variation of it, as follows:

"I love and accept myself whether or not I _____

_____"

(...I pass this test, get this job or promotion, my partner praises or criticizes me, etc).

Games provide a lot of stimulation and excitement, but they also produce negative payoffs that leave us wondering what happened and why some part of our lives is not working. They also further our negative life story, so that though we spend so much energy struggling to have positive outcomes, all the while, outside of our awareness, we are setting up the negative outcomes, the heart attack, the stroke, the broken relationship, for example, that will lead to the big negative payoff of our life story.

# AUTHORING OUR OWN LIFE STORY

*There is no agony like bearing an untold story inside of you.*

Maya Angelou

We all endure pain and wounding in our lives; it is part of the human condition. But when we have not repaired and healed these injuries, we have to manage them. And rooted as they are in the stages of our cyclic unfolding, we attempt to manage them by placing ourselves at odds with how we're designed. We fight this cyclic, ever—evolving process, creating for ourselves the single most significant reason we run into trouble in our personal lives. And denying this process in ourselves or in others is the single most important reason we sabotage our relationships.

When we first combat, then deny our inner process and the work of its stages, we attempt to place our own wounds into a great and impersonal story, thus giving weight to them. As poet Robert Bly points out, we elevate them into "mythological space" where they "fit into a great and impersonal story" or script.[26]

But the way we were as children does not go away when we get older, for our entire personal history is recorded in our extra—genetic programming and manifested through our ego states, a dynamic part of us motivating our current experiences. If we did not get what we needed to conclude unfinished business and heal completely, we continue to seek it symbolically through dramatic scenes we enact in our present life, unconsciously acting out scenes from our "script," where our personal collection of early decisions and unmet needs, pain, trauma and the decisions we made about them are kept but now long forgotten. Outside of our awareness, our script continues to program our current experiences.[33] Scripts represent our attempts to get needs met that were not met originally. When we play out our script as grownups, we act in ways that are symbolic of the original painful and unsatisfactory experience. Thus, script behavior is predetermined. We are controlled by yesterday, as if haunted by demons or hunted by witches. We are just the opposite of spontaneous, autonomous, creative beings. Prisoners of our past, we are not free to live today.

How our scripts affect our relationships is easy to understand. Imagine, for example, how our lives might unfold if we are unconsciously playing out the Little Red Riding Hood story in our adult life. We will symbolically act out dramas involving getting sent on errands (somebody else is responsible for what we're doing and we are innocent, i.e., daydreaming instead of paying attention); going through "the woods" (dark, dangerous places with no protection); we are accosted while innocently doing a good deed; our life story is filled with predators who find us because they are searching for someone who's "checked out" and therefore vulnerable; etc., and we even take a turn at being predatory ourselves.

Or consider our fate if we are unconsciously playing out the myth of Sisyphus, who was condemned by the gods to a life of futile labor, ceaselessly rolling a stone up a mountain only to have it roll down again, whereupon he would have to start over. In this script we continually reenter hopeless situations (discounting our own power), then when the symbolic "stone" of life rolls down again, we sigh and commence the whole absurd undertaking all over again. The "stone" we push up the hill may take on a variety of forms——new business ventures, for example, or a series of new relationships in which we entertain the false belief that "things will be different this time." But they will not be different, because we have already doomed ourselves to failure. Typically this is because we are so terrified of exercising our own right to choose that we consider a hopeless repetition of fruitless effort to be better than the consequences that might befall us should we take our own power; and all of this takes place quite out of our awareness.

Most of us did not get everything we needed as we were growing up, so most of us have scripts. We are attached to some aspects of our personal history in the present moment. Using script programs we structure our time by symbolically attempting to meet the needs we had yesterday or yesteryear. These symbolic efforts do not work, however, because they suffer from bad timing. Still, we may continue the same unrewarding and repetitious patterns because our needs remain unmet.

Although there are many varieties of script programs, they all function to make us seem some way other than we really are. We are not being ourselves, true to our own emotional nature. Yet what happened to us is not who we are, which is really good news. It means that the process of becoming free of our script limitations is the route back to becoming ourselves——becoming who we really are. This process is the progression covered stage by stage in Part Two.

Each particular illusion is one we decided to assume as we were growing up, in order to get the caring that was available.

Below is a summary of our conditions when we've decided to fight and deny our internal cyclical process:

**Stay Little**
**(Don't Grow Up)**

Our parents may not actually have said "Stay little," but they may have communicated it because they were afraid of our growing up and leaving them.

The way we get strokes is to look little and inadequate.

We act as if the only way to do things is to get someone else to do them for us.

We try to keep close to people.

**Hurry and Grow Up**
**(Don't Be Dependent)**

Our parents may not actually have said, "Don't be little," but they may have communicated it because they feared close contact and dependency.

The way we get strokes is by acting threatening.

We act as if the only way to do things is to do them our way only.

We try to keep people at a distance.

| | |
|---|---|
| We are controlled by the space around us. | We control the space around us. |
| We diminish our awareness to look impotent. | We heighten our awareness to look powerful. |
| We try to "kill time." | We try to "make time." |
| We have trouble making up our minds, often waiting for someone else to make them up for us. | We point out other people's faults a lot. We are among the first to notice others' imperfections. |
| We rarely get mad; often acting scared instead. | We rarely get scared. We deny our fear and get mad instead. |
| We agree with people often, no matter what they are saying, unless they say, "Disagree!" | We act in opposition to most situations; we don't often agree with others. |
| We try to anticipate what others need before they ask. | We are afraid to let other people know we have needs. |
| We take care of other people, even when we don't feel like it. | We are afraid to take care of other people because we feel we'll get "milked dry." |

The beginning of getting out of our script is recognizing that we are in it. Recognition is the first step. The second step is identifying the need that our script attempts to meet, however unsuccessfully. We have then started to let go of yesterday's pain and to be alive today.

# THE CYCLE OF LIFE

**Activities for Scripts**

1. Return to the lists above and check each aspect that applies to you.

2. Think of the child you once were. Who is the older friend or relative that child most closely identified with?

_____

3. Describe in a sentence or two the positive aspects of that person's life:

_____

The negative aspects:

_____

4. Think about your life now. In what ways are you following a life pattern similar to this person?

_____

5. What was your favorite fairy tale as a child?

_____

6. Think for a moment about any negative or harmful patterns you still play out in your current life. If you continue on your present course, where will you be...

In 5 years: _____

In 10 years: _____

In 20 years: _____

7. What do you need to do now to turn that negative script payoff into a positive desirable one?

_____

_____

# TRANSFORMATION

*Change your life today. Don't gamble on the future, act now, without delay.*

Simone de Beauvoir

Transformation is the inner process through which we release ourselves from the confines of our script beliefs so that we can center our selves back into the evolving stages of our lives. Thus we live out the meaning of the word "transform," because we change in structure, form, condition, nature or character. Our transformation parallels the metamorphosis of the caterpillar, which enters its cocoon only to exit as a butterfly.

This internal revolution begins when we turn from denying our pain to facing it, ready to give it full acknowledgment, to provide however much energy and attention is needed for a resolution.

Everything we need to know about our stuck places and how to heal them exists within them as part of our original "recording."[34] By turning to face such places where we have been trapped, we align ourselves to access this information. We gradually become more conscious of what happened, how we feel about it, and what we need to do to heal and free ourselves. As we begin to become aware that we can heal, we slowly begin to tear down the wall between our current limited selves and our essential wholeness.

We can release ourselves from the limits of script beliefs whether they were made the day we were born, weaned, toilet trained, punished for truancy, on our first date, abused by a partner, or injured in a war. We can transform the limiting beliefs of our life story no matter when they were acquired. For example, if in our original experience of emotional distress we decided we have no right to exist, we can reenter that experience with the light of our presence and consciousness today. We can release any dammed—up energy and emerge with full support for our right to exist. We have then moved from opposing our basic emotional nature to being supported by it.

The roots of our original pain, issues and decisions that still bind us today can reach all the way back to the beginning of our lives. That is because we program our personalities as we build them during all the stages of our childhood. Such codes are contained in our extra—genetic learning system, made originally from the interactions we have with others while we are undergoing our natural process of development. They now function in our grown—up life just like the automatic pilot in an airplane——as encoded messages that automatically tell us how to run things. If our programming is faulty, we may have a rough flight or even a crash landing. In such a case, we can redesign the program to support the workings of our personalities and bodies.

The place to start when encountering problems in our outer life is to go inside ourselves. This may seem counterintuitive at first. After all, if there's a problem in the outer world, why would we then turn within to seek its solution? The answer is both simple and profound: we are powerful beings who are always in the process of manifesting our beliefs, however unaware we may be of what they are or that we are doing it. This reality is borne out not only in the world of counseling and therapy, but also in the worlds of quantum physics, brain research and understanding of neuropeptides. All confirm that what's going on inside us is far more important in shaping the contents of our lives than are any outer events.

How can this work? In quantum terms, we interact with the outside world, provoking the outside world to coalesce into a particular state. It is a truth four—year—olds know well, for they are still living in their magical state, where they are grappling with the idea that if they entertain certain thoughts, they make them come true. They know, as we have forgotten, that we are participating in creating the effects of reality.

Brain and neuropeptide research have added to the picture begun by quantum physics. To summarize, they report that when we are in a particular state of consciousness, we think a thought, and that concentrated piece of information becomes matter. We have, in essence, turned waves into particles with our attention, thus bringing them into being in the pattern of our thought.[35]

However, we cannot simply delete such instructions now. We need to encode new ones to replace the old. To develop new encoding we require new interactions with others while carrying out the same tasks of development.  Then we not only write new and healthy programming, we also receive external support from contact with others.  This also supports us in maintaining our connection to reality, and helps prevent us from getting stuck in self—destructive spaces.  This is a process greatly aided by listening to new stories——those from others as well as myths and fairy tales——for they contain prescriptive tasks we can carry out to transform our inner lives.

Since most destructive programs at least imply that some aspect of our self is crazy, we may feel as if we were about to go crazy as we venture closer to a solution.  If we have spent our lives up until now perched on a powder key of archaic rage, we have no doubt been careful not to light any emotional matches.  Our decision to turn and face that anger will probably not be made without some resistance.  A wee small voice inside us may object, "No, no! I'll kill somebody," or "No, no! Somebody will kill me!"

This is a good time to remember that whether we live out of our collection of illusions or out of our basic sanity is our choice, *our* decision.  If we don't keep this fact in mind, we may prevent ourselves from continuing our process of emotional transformation, to avoid experiencing this often intense fear of going crazy.  When we are ready to become aware of beliefs formerly held outside of our conscious program, we are beginning to position ourselves to rewrite our beliefs.  The outcome of our journey depends on whether we want to work out unfinished business responsibly or act it out without being aware of doing so. It is our decision alone. And, we can arrange protection to make the process safe.

The following is a structure for beginning the process of transformation by naming the aspects of the dynamic that are revealed on the surface. Then the next chapter presents a way to identify these beliefs in such a way that the seeds of the solution are revealed even as we are discovering the problem.

# The Cycle of Life

**Activities to Begin Transformation**

1. Feeling "crazy" is a response to an experience which we believe is not okay or is abnormal, or in which we're set up to make a choice in which no matter how we choose, we lose (referred to as a double bind).

From the following list, circle the feelings or experiences that you learned were "not okay," bad, or abnormal.

| | | | |
|---|---|---|---|
| ____joyful | ____sad | ____tired | ____grieved |
| ____proud | ____energetic | ____sexy | ____doubtful |
| ____mad | ____jealous | ____aggressive | ____glad |
| ____scared | ____hungry | ____timid | ____full |

Other: _____

2. For each item you circled above, describe what you do to avoid having that experience. For example:

Instead of feeling *mad, I get scared.*

Instead of feeling *scared, I get busy doing things.*

Instead of feeling _____ I _____

Instead of feeling _____ I _____

Instead of feeling _____ I _____

Instead of feeling _____ I _____

Instead of feeling _____ I _____

3. Now read the list again. This time, next to each item you circled, place a number on a scale of 1 to 10 to denote the level of resistance

you feel about allowing yourself to feel this experience, with number 1 being the lowest and 10 being the highest. This number represents the degree of protection you may need to arrange for the transformation which will allow the experience to be okay, healthy and normal again.

# IDENTIFYING SELF—SABOTAGE

*Friendship with oneself is all—important, because without it one cannot be friends with anyone else in the world.*

Eleanor Roosevelt

We have already begun to free ourselves from relentlessly reenacting the beliefs in our scripts when we own that we have unfinished business, even if we do not know what it is. Without this step, all the others that lead to our freedom and satisfaction remain inaccessible.

Disowning our unfinished business negatively affects our relationships because we unconsciously set up others to carry what we disown. We angle to get others to carry our emotional "hot potato."[36] In other words, we have passed our emotional issue to someone else who carries it for us and may also act it out for us. In so doing, we place our own internal emotional conflicts, troubles and pain into the external environment of our relationships. Then we think our relationship is not working because of the other person. This can lead to a series of relationships that all end up the same. We are constantly trying to manage or get rid of the person expressing the problem instead of looking to ourselves to see what we might be passing on to others.

Our investment in disowning our emotional issues results from the belief that they are so powerful/ painful/ damaging/ horrible that we won't be able to stand becoming conscious of them. Therefore one of the most important steps we can take in working through the emotional issues that underlie our scripts is deciding that we can indeed stand what we are feeling.

We believe we can't stand facing these issues because inside we are still responding to a trauma as if it were happening now——as if it were a real and present danger. Actually, though, the feeling of danger is archaic. In other words, it is from somewhere in our past, where it remains unexpressed, unresolved, perhaps because it was dangerous to feel or express in the situation in which it originally occurred.

When as adults we decide to get in touch with and be aware of these feelings, our internal survival reaction can kick in. It's as if in our brain and body we believe we are going to destroy our family or its current equivalent——our friends, families, work situation or organization to which we belong. But in fact, we are merely re—experiencing a previous danger. The feeling of danger is part of our old program, an illusion carried over from yesteryear.

Next, we need to deal with feeling fragile. We continue to feel fragile and impotent as adults because as children we gave up our power in the original situation in order to maintain safety and stability. In the original situation we avoided completing the emotional work we needed to do because it would have threatened our safety. In other words, in the original situation it made perfect sense, emotionally speaking, to put our emotional needs on hold. But now the idea that finishing this emotional business will again create danger is part of our old script illusion, our archaic feelings. It is not current reality——unless we act out the problem instead of working it out.

## Identifying Self—Sabotage

Having decided to experience what we are feeling, getting clear that we are not too fragile to cope, and preparing to complete our emotional business responsibly instead of acting it out, we can keep the illusion in clearer perspective. We see it for what it is——just an old piece of unfinished business——and we see ourselves for who we are: powerful and capable.

We are now ready to discover what exactly it is we've put on "hold." Rather than being a scary or upsetting process, it can actually prove to be exciting. We are about to find out how self—sabotaging behavior in our current life actually makes perfect sense when seen from the perspective of the emotional logic of our attempts to protect ourselves from further harm.

Identifying a script issue means deciding to think about it. The following is a way of structuring our thinking about our unfinished emotional business. In picking up paper and pencil, we aid our thinking, our Adult computing processes. Use the method below to put together the pieces of information as they become conscious. Placing them within this structure reveals the entire dynamic of the issue in such a way that what the solution will look like is identified as well.

Identifying the unfinished business that drives our script is always a process of trial and error. Therefore we may need to change the entries in the blanks several times as we focus our feelings and can gauge more accurately what feels right.

## Activities for Identifying Problems

The following is a way to identify this total picture of both our personal issue and the direction for its resolution. Complete the first five lines of the Structure for Thinking, composing them in any order. When they are finished, go on to the next two to complete your Blueprint for Healing. When you've concluded those, fill in the last one, keeping in mind that any image that involves injury to oneself or others is not a healing image. When such an image arises, go back and keep repeating the two lines of your Blueprint for Healing until you arrive at an image that represents being truly free of the issue you've identified. You will know you have found it when you automatically breathe a big sigh of relief when mentally picturing the image.

### Structure for Thinking [37]

I am _____

(*feeling*)

because I think that if I _____

(*behavior I initiate*)

I will be _____

(*unhealthy Parental response*)

instead of _____

(*healthy Parental response*)

So I _____

(*problem justifying behaviors, games*)

IDENTIFYING SELF—SABOTAGE

## Blueprint for Healing[38]

I _____

(insert the information from Line Two above)

and I am _____

(insert the information from Line Four above)


## Healing Image

When I repeat the affirming message to myself, the following healing image comes to mind: _____

(describe in words, or draw)


The following are two examples of emotional problems using this structure:

### Structure for Thinking

| | |
|---|---|
| I am | scared |
| | (*feeling*) |
| because I think that if I | cry to be held |
| | (*behavior I initiate*) |
| I will be | beaten |
| | (*unhealthy Parental response*) |
| instead of | nurtured |
| | (*healthy Parental response*) |
| so I | act cute and coy when I need something, wait to ask until I can't stand it, drink to numb the need, smoke and eat |
| | (*problem justifying behavior*) |

# The Cycle of Life

## Blueprint for Healing

I <u>cry to be held</u>
(information from Line Two above)

and I am <u>nurtured</u>
(information from Line Four above)

## Healing Image

When I repeat the affirming message to myself, the following healing image comes to mind:

<u>floating in the warm waters of a blue lagoon, being rocked by the waves while my head is being massaged</u>
(describe in words, or draw)

******

## Structure for Thinking

I am <u>angry</u>
*(feeling)*

because I think that if I <u>show any angry behavior at all</u>
*(behavior I initiate)*

I will be <u>abandoned because my parents get sick and hysterical</u>
*(unhealthy Parental response)*

instead of <u>being, stayed with and calmly supported to deal with my anger</u>
*(healthy Parental response)*

So I <u>act scared, helpless, weak and fragile, and do what others want me to do</u>
*(problem justifying behavior)*

## Identifying Self—Sabotage

### Blueprint for Healing

I <u>　　show my anger　　　　　　　　　　　　　　　</u>
　　　(information from Line Two above)

And I am <u>stayed with and calmly supported to deal with my anger</u>
　　　　　　　　　　　　　　　　　　　　(information from

　　　　　　　　　　　　　　　　　　　　Line Four above)

### Healing Image

When I repeat the affirming message to myself, the following healing image comes to mind: ____expressing my rage while surrounded by my parents and family who calmly receive my feelings, apologize, offer me a drink of water, wash my tears away and hold me
_____

(describe in words, or draw)


Think about a difficulty you are experiencing in your current life. Fill out the following *Structure for Thinking*.

Fill out Line One using the words a five—year—old would use for feelings, such as scared, mad, sad and glad.

For Line Two, be specific about what *developmental stage task* is most associated with the feeling. In turn, this will offer accurate clues as to the archaic age of the problem. Use the following list to aid that process:

## Developmental Stage Tasks

### Stage One

Be rather than do, build or renew sustaining emotional connections with others, be touched and have intimate physical contact, gather strength (often by asking others to take over for a while), take in, be nourished, be recharged.

### Stage Two

Explore the environment without having to think about it; develop sensory awareness by doing; taste, touch, smell, feel, hear and see what the world is about; feel the earth, find footing, get in touch with the ground; seek a variety of stimulation; be free to move out into the world, to follow our own urges.

### Stage Three

Find out our importance in relation to others; develop concepts, take in information and learn to think; find our limits and those of the world; make connections between sensory events; express negativity and ambivalence; push against others; have what's mine apart from yours; exert our opinion; test reality.

### Stage Four

Find out "Who am I?" and create an identity, discover what being male or female means, test definitions of reality through consequences, exert power to affect relationships, separate fantasy from reality, develop the ability to organize and change our internal reality.

### Stage Five

Experiment with different ways of doing things; develop physical, intellectual, emotional and social skills; argue, hassle and disagree;

# IDENTIFYING SELF—SABOTAGE

exclude others' methods until we make our own; learn new morals, manners or values; make mistakes to find out what works.

**Stage Six**

Integrate sexuality with needs from other stages, grow beyond our parenting (or mentoring) relationship, develop our own personal philosophy, develop as a sexually mature person, revisit each earlier stage and update it if necessary, develop a place among grownups, prepare to succeed in the world as a grownup.

In Line Three, describe what you anticipate is going to happen if you truly carry out the tasks you listed in Line Two.

For Line Four, use the juiciest, most wonderful words you can think of to describe the hoped—for response that would make you melt inside just to think of it.

The contents of Line Five are often the first ones we become aware of, for they are our defenses. For example, we may start to fill out the structure, only to become distracted, want to eat, light a cigarette, have a drink, remember a wrong and yell at the offender, feel too tired because we're overworked, etc. So notice the reactions you have as you begin, and for each one, name it and place it in Line Five. You will quickly have a complete list of the defensive behaviors you've employed to avoid what you are now working to identify.

## Structure for Thinking

I feel _____

(feeling)

because I think that if I _____

(behavior I initiate. Note: Use list above to guide/ inspire you)

I will be _____

(unhealthy response)

instead of _____

(healthy response)

so I _____

(problem justifying behavior, games)

## Blueprint for Healing

I _____

(insert the information from Line Two above)

and I am _____

(insert the information from Line Four above)

## Healing Image

When I repeat the affirming message to myself, the following healing image comes to mind: _____

(describe in words, or draw)

## IDENTIFYING SELF—SABOTAGE

1. Return to the five—line emotional issue identified above and review it to appreciate the emotional wisdom it reveals. Answer the following:

   a. How much are my current relationships based on my doing Line Five? _____

   b. Out of all the times I relate to people, how often do I get Line Three responses from them? _____

   c. When I actually do the behavior in Line Two, what response do I get from others? _____

   d. How do these responses match the ones I really want? _____

2. Re—read the sentence you have just completed in 1. Allowing yourself to be creative, and without censoring any idea, no matter how absurd or impossible, list all the things you might do about it. (For example, one person who completed a Structure for Thinking about money worries made this list: see a therapist, skip town, refuse to pay any of my bills, insist that someone else handle it, borrow money, regress to an age too young to be expected to deal with it, consult with an accountant, pay part of each bill, pay all of some bills and delay payment on others.)

   a. _____
   b. _____
   c. _____
   d. _____
   e. _____

f. _____

g. _____

h. _____

i. _____

3. Without *thinking* about it, write down how old you feel when you experience the problem you identified above.

I feel _____ (months, years) old

Use this age as a reference in choosing which stage in Part Two applies to this issue, and therefore which tasks are involved and what kind of support for resolution is needed, consistent with that stage.

# PROTECTION

*Why, you're nothing but a pack of cards!*

Alice, in <u>Alice in Wonderland</u>

If we encounter great resistance in attempting to identify the roots of self—sabotage, that is an indication that we need more protection.[39] Creating protection means setting things up so we feel safe to progress further, without causing any injury or harm to ourselves, anyone else or the environment. Protection clears the path ahead so we can feel whatever we feel and stay conscious in the face of those feelings. It is the key with which we can open up the door to our vast storehouse of past experiences.

Protection is essential on our journey into these spaces because they are beyond the influence of the usual states of consciousness which contain our counterscript. A counterscript is a collection of methods we have learned to use to temporarily neutralize or to "counter" our destructive script. Protection provides an external environment in which we can not only prevent danger, but also permanently resolve the script.

When we are protected, we have eliminated any immediate danger of injury or loss that will result from our facing the challenge of uncovering the source of self—sabotage. The particular protection needed will be unique to each person. As we set up protection in each situation we can keep in mind three central guidelines:

1. We need protection in a form specific to the age of the inner Child who made the script decision. If the decision was made in our teenage years, we can receive others' compassion through words. That same compassion must be translated into direct physical contact to connect with our inner Child, who is younger than words.

2. To feel protected enough to work through script issues successfully, we require right here and now one or more caring, competent people. We need to feel secure enough to let out into our consciousness a part of ourselves who may be scared, sad, angry or hurting. To make sure others' support is real and not just talk, we need to grant them the right to say "No" to anything they may not want to do. Such protection contributes to a successful outcome because their discomfort sheds new light on the entire situation.

3. We create protection with others by making agreements. Such contracts are the vehicle through which we give and receive protection.[40] In Adult language a contract is a legal, mutual agreement entered into by one or more competent parties. It states clearly what each person wants from the relationship and what each person is going to give. In Child words, a contract creates safe methods for giving and receiving love.

We can make profound changes when we focus our external relationships in this way. First we become aware that a present destructive pattern is a repetition of an earlier traumatic experience. Then by arranging the protection needed to resolve the earlier experience, we create a new experience that by its very existence has begun to replace the original one. We feel safer and stronger as each moment passes.

## The Cycle of Life

**Activities for Protection**

1. When I think about arranging protection for the little girl or boy inside of me, I feel:

_____

2. The little girl or boy inside me needs protection from (circle those that apply):

   a.   Being physically hurt
   b.   Being emotionally hurt
   c.   Being criticized
   d.   Being blamed
   e.   Having to take care of others by growing up too fast
   f.   Having to take care of others by not growing up
   g.   Being abandoned
   h.   Being unloved
   i.   Feeling unworthy

Include items circled above when you make a contract with others for protection. Following is an example of such a contract:[41]

PROTECTION

**Contract for Protection**

1. I will stop:

_____

_____

_____

(from the Structure for Thinking, Line Five)

2. I will start:

_____

_____

_____

(from the *Structure for Thinking*, Line Two)

3. And when I do, I need you to:

_____

_____

_____

(from the Structure for Thinking, Line Four)

4. Underlying issue:

_____

_____

(That doing the behavior entered in the Structure for Thinking, Line Two will cause Line Three to happen).

## The Cycle of Life

**Bracketing**

Before starting to work, it is important to review guidelines for bracketing the issue you are working on so it does not bleed over into your life outside the environment in which you are doing your emotional work.

Bracketing is a process to support staying grown—up instead of regressing. It means containing emotional issues so we can work them out in an appropriate setting instead of acting them out in everyday life. It is important for us to bracket because it protects us from the unwanted consequences of toxic emotional spills in our current lives. It honors the fact that working out emotionally stuck places can take special circumstances——ones that deal with those places in a protected structure where we have a specific contract to do so. When we bracket issues, we set them aside until the proper time and situation in which the protection we need is in place.

*How to Bracket*

1. Picture the Child part of you who needs to deal with a personal issue. Then picture giving that Child to some safe person to take care of until you get to the situation (counseling, therapy, recovery group, workshop, etc.) where you can do the work.

2. Tell that Child that you, the grownup, are making an absolute commitment and will arrange for a time and place that is safe so the Child can do the healing work.

## PROTECTION

3. So that the Child will trust you, make those arrangements now or as soon as possible.

4. Tell your Child when that time will be (for example, no later than two weeks from now).

5. Visualize hugging your Child and putting it in a safe place.

6. Use your other ego states to get back out of your Child part, e.g., think, enjoy some grownup fun, etc.

7. If your Child part peeks through again from time to time, tell it that you know it is there, you hear it; remind it of your commitment and explain that this is not the right time to do the healing work you need to do.

8. Tell your Child to cooperate with the grown—up part so the grownup can get what is needed and not be sabotaged.

9. In the proper time and place, with proper protection and in cooperation with your grownup, let your Child do the necessary healing work. During this time, do not allow interference by your grown—up self with its grown—up concerns.

10. Write on a piece of paper the issue(s) you are bracketing for right now. Use the following to help you state this:

a. With regard to the problem I want to resolve, I am feeling _____

_____

b. I feel this in my body (describe *where* you feel it) _____

_____

c. I feel _____ (months, years) old.

## The Cycle of Life

    d. What I do *not* want you to do is _____

_____

(Examples: Leave me, criticize me, tell me to be quiet, etc.)

    e. What I know so far about what I will want you to do is _____

_____

Examples: Touch my head, tell me it's okay to scream, give me a pillow to hit, etc.)

    f. When I resolve this, what I will be able to have or do in my life is (describe): _____

_____

11. Fold the paper, then on the outside write the date and time you will deal with it.

12. Put the paper away, and as you do so, reaffirm your commitment to maintaining this bracketing.

*****

The "Resources" section at the end of this book provides some sources of support for undertaking this kind of inner work.

# RECLAIMING OUR ESSENTIAL SELVES

*It is better to conquer yourself than to win a thousand battles. Then the victory is yours. It cannot be taken from you, not by angels or by demons, heaven or hell.*

Buddha

We know a great deal about the process of freeing ourselves from our inner emotionally stuck places and freeing ourselves to emerge into the ground of our real emotional selves: sane and healthy. This knowledge has been gathered from the experiences of thousands of people around the world working in a variety of settings. These include individual counseling and therapy, personal growth marathons, workshops, seminars, consciousness—raising groups, group therapy meetings and addiction recovery programs.

Distilling information from all these sources reveals some commonalities for a successful process and a successful outcome. Here is one such distillation in the form of a useful set of guidelines:

1. Participation by all parties concerned is voluntary. There is no force or coercion of any kind.

2. All parties agree to be mutually supportive, not critical or abusive. This means dealing with negative feelings in a straightforward and honest manner.

3. The emotional atmosphere is informal, relaxed and personal.

4. The physical atmosphere is comfortable and casual.

5. Non—sexual physical contact is appropriate as long as each person agrees to this.

6. There are good boundaries for the physical space so the work at hand is not bothered by distractions such as other people marching through or phones ringing and being answered. Such various interruptions are put on hold.

7. The group as a whole has well—established meeting time boundaries with an agreed—upon start and end time.

8. So there is enough time for all the people who want to work, each individual has a start and stop time that is mutually agreed on.

9. The work being done can be specific to the age of the Child who is still experiencing the emotional trauma, shock or disturbance.

10. The person working is able to bracket——to work on the emotional issue during the time allotted but not carry it over into their work lives, marriages, parenting, etc.

11. When starting their work, the person offers a brief description of the work he or she wishes to do. This includes information from their Structure for Thinking, Blueprint for Healing, and Contract so that the other person or people are clear about what the person needs to do and wants from others, including the nature of a resolution.

For example: "I have a pain in my stomach. I think I've been swallowing anger most of my life. I think it's young because I feel wobbly when I let the feeling rise, and I have pain in my teeth, maybe teething pain. I will probably need you to give me something to bite. I think I had to give up stroking when I was active. That's probably why I'm angry. I want a lot of stroking from people, especially when I'm active. That's how I'll know I don't have to give up other needs in order to *do* things."

So far there have not been any needs that are actually unmeetable. There have been no archaic problems that have turned out to be unsolvable. No piece of suffering has been so large or severe or scary that it could not be released or resolved. People have been able to look at the facts and say, "I can solve it. It is solvable."[42]

As we go through the process of going "sane," we return to the way we truly are made emotionally. We come back to our fundamental emotional sanity, our essential selves. We set ourselves free to live in the ever—evolving progression of our cyclic nature.

# CONCLUSION
## In the End is the Beginning

*To be awake is to be alive!*

Henry David Thoreau

To turn toward our cyclic, evolving self and synchronize with our own inner, swirling stream of life is to restore ourselves to harmony within ourselves and with all of nature. As we accept that we evolve in a cyclic pattern our entire lives, we settle in, become more centered and able to have a deeper, more grounded and more natural relationship with ourselves. We free ourselves from major internal pressure as we end our war with how we're made. We develop inner peace as we become receptive to our own inner changes, for we know we are living in harmony with the natural laws that underlie how we are designed. We embody nature's rhythms as our own. We become increasingly stable inside ourselves. Gradually, we come to rest in this regularization, relieved at last from the effort of maintaining ourselves on the shifting foundations of our own illusions. With each turning and each stage we become more fully ourselves.

Then we are able both to rise to the challenges and accept the gifts of each stage.

In Stage One we are challenged to begin again, to enter new territory, to face the unknown, while we accept the gifts of being given time, an opportunity to regroup, catch our developmental breath, update our trust relationships, tune in to ourselves, reorganize our relationships to be in tune with our needs in this new cycle that stretches before us.

In Stage Two we stretch out into a world that has become somehow new, unknown. We have to feel our way along via our sensory pathways, exploring to see what's out there while still maintaining those life—sustaining bonds we established in Stage One.

In Stage Three we work to establish ourselves as separate beings, becoming temporarily oppositional and contrary, wanting to be different than others, gathering information, testing, learning to think in new ways.

In Stage Four we revisit our old roles, our former identities, shedding old "selves" like clothes that no longer fit, while searching our social world to establish ourselves anew in updated roles and relationships.

In Stage Five, we strive to add the skills we will need to carry out our newly established, updated self. What do we need to know how to do? What do we value now, from this perspective?

And in Stage Six, we bring all these changes together, forging them into one complete whole, becoming ready to break away from our familiar dependencies into a new life, whereupon we repeat the round again..

As we repeat the stages, we can decide to use them to accomplish our life goals. If we choose not to use them, we will merely repeat the past with all its limiting familiarity. If instead we employ this opportunity to create the results we want in life, we enter into the vast, endless process of growth, merging with the creative potential of the universe that is our birthright. We then feel connected and alive, for we are creating our own vision for how to live. We are pursuing our own dreams instead of someone else's illusions.

As we continue to return through the stages, if we pay attention to liberating ourselves from the self—limiting beliefs of our past, our contact with the basic truths of life expands, and we discover that:

The cycle is the vessel of our lives but it's not who we are;

We grow through stages but are not our stages;

We have a life story but are not our story;

We have and release limiting beliefs but are not our beliefs;

We are something beyond all that.

In our revolving journey we are evolving from being a child of our parents to a child of the universe. We develop spontaneity, playfulness, joy. We are more fully alive, fully ourselves, more wise, capable of both rewarding intimacy and life—sustaining personal boundaries. Increasingly integrated inside, we discover a lightness of being, a fundamental good humor, and we feel connected both to ourselves and to "it all."

We may be '"captives on a carousel of time," we may live our lives in this spiraling cycle, but that doesn't mean that is who we are. It is simply what we are undergoing in this earthly sojourn. So, then, who are we, beyond this process? William Wordsworth implied an answer to that question when he wrote

## The Cycle of Life

*Not in entire forgetfulness,*
*And not in utter nakedness,*
*But trailing clouds of glory do we come*
*From God, who is our home:*
*Heaven lies about us in our infancy!*[43]

The Christian disciple Paul, writing in I Corinthians put it even more directly when he said,

> "Know ye not that ye are the temple of God, and that the Spirit of God dwelleth in you? [44]

Discovering that we are conscious beings on a journey through a material world, spiritual beings in a time—bound physical body, what does this mean about how we can best live our lives? Again the poets serve as prophets, divining wise counsel. From the East, the voice of the ancients echoes through the ages:

> *With this great understanding of the end and the beginning, and of how the six stages are accomplished (each according to its own time), the Sage mounts them as though they were six dragons, and heads for heaven.*
>
> Tuan—chuan
> *I Ching, Book of Changes*

CONCLUSION

# Resources

For a complete guide to the Cycle of Development and the stages, see *Cycles of Power: A User's Guide to the Seven Seasons of Life*, Pamela Levin, published by The Nourishing Company.

For the French language version, *Les Cycles de L'Identite, Comment se developpent nos competences tout au long de notre vie*, InterEditions, Paris France, 2000, go to nourishingcompany.com or

http://dunod.com/pages/ouvrages/ficheouvrage.asp?id=48878

For a variety of articles on emotional and physical health improvement, visit www.nourishingcompany.com.

Pamela Levin's books on physical health improvement include *Perfect Bones: A Six—point Plan for Healthy Bones,* Celestial Arts, Berkeley, Ca. 2002, and *The Female Hormone Journey:; Lifetime Care of Your Hormones*, The Nourishing Company, Ukiah, 2005. They are available on the web at perfectbones.com, femalehormonejourney.com

For referral to mental health professionals, organizational consultants or educators familiar with the concepts presented here, contact The International Transactional Analysis Association, where you may obtain a list of members in good standing in your area. See itaa—neg.org or

The International Transactional Analysis Association

2186 Rheem Drive #B—1

Pleasanton, CA 94588

Phone: 1—925/600—8110

***Transactional Analysis Organizations***

The entire world list of TA organizations can be accessed at http://itaa—net.org/community/comm.htm

The following are relevant to English language speakers:

USATAA — United States of America Transactional Analysis Association.

www.usataa.org

Southeast Institute www.seinstitute.com USA USATAA

www.usataa.org

International Transactional Analysis Association

A scientific organization which facilitates international communication.

www.itaa—net.org

European Association of Transactional Analysis

The European Association of Transactional Analysis is a membership organization for European TA training organizations.

www.eatanews.org

Western Pacific Association of Transactional Analysis (WPATA)

# Resources

www.wpata.com.au

| | |
|---|---|
| In Canada: The Change Institute | www.thechangeinstitute.ca |
| Eastwind Institute | www.eastwindinstitute.com |
| Touchstone Counselling | www.touchstonecounselling.ca |
| In England: The Berne Institute | www.theberne.com |
| Elan in Manchester | www.mantra.demon.co.uk |
| Institute of Transactional Analysis (ITA) | www.ita.org.uk |
| Manchester Institute | www.mcpt.co.uk |
| The Metanoia Institute | www.metanoia.ac.uk |

In Ireland: Transactional Analysis in Ireland (TAI)
    http://homepage.eircom.net/~liztai37

In New Zealand: Auckland TA Training Institute (ATATI)
    www.atati.co.nz

New Zealand Transactional Analysis Association (NZTAA)
    www.nztaa.org.nz

Lucy Mackie <mackie.fam@clear.net.nz>

Wellington Transactional Analysis Training Institute
    www.hewitt.gen.nz/

## *Addiction Recovery Support*

Addiction Recovery Guide: Your Internet Guide to Recovery

Recovery resources for drug and alcohol addiction and abuse, including 12—step and holistic approaches. Also a message board with support forums for pain.

www.addictionrecoveryguide.org

Drug Recovery Support Addiction Recovery Support Groups. Locate A Meeting In Your Area!
www.Unhooked.com

## *Therapists*

See the Transactional Analysis organizations above, and

Find—a—Therapist.com —— Find a Therapist, Psychologist International directory and referral service containing personalized listings of therapists and mental health professionals.

www.find—a—therapist.com

Find A Therapist

Browse an Extensive Directory of U.S. Therapists at *PsychologyToday*. www.PsychologyToday.com

Find A Therapist Who doesn't just say "Uh huh" and "How do you feel about that?" www.WomensPsychotherapy.com

## *Pre— and Perinatal Work*

Association for Pre— & Perinatal Psychology and Health (APPPAH) For therapists who specialize in pre— and perinatal trauma work.
www.birthpsychology.com

# Glossary

**ADAPTED**  A fixed pattern of behavior designed to please others or one's own internal Parent.

**ARCHAIC**  Old; arising from an earlier stage of development, often in childhood.

**BRACKETING**  Restricting issues to be worked on to appropriate times and places where protection is provided.

**CONTAMINATION**  The clouding of a present experience by an unintegrated past experience so that what happens now is felt to be the same as the past event.

**CONTRACT**  A legal, mutual agreement entered into by two or more competent parties; a vehicle through which we give and receive protection.

**COUNTERSCRIPT**  A collection of messages which can temporarily neutralize destructive extra—genetic script patterns.

**CYCLE**  A recurring period of time, especially one in which certain events repeat themselves in the same order and intervals.

**DISCOUNT**  To refuse to take into account; to devalue, especially through not recognizing a person or a problem and not acknowledging the problem's importance, ability to solve it or the fact that it can be solved.

**EGO STATE** State of the self when transacting. Named Parent, Adult and Child by Eric Berne, they provide the foundation for analyzing transactions.

**ESCALATE** To increase the energy in a feeling or problem until it is out of proportion.

**GAME** A series of ulterior transactions beginning with a discount, followed by a switch in roles and ending with a payoff that justifies, rather than solves, a problem, as used in Transactional Analysis.

**INJUNCTION** Parental messages that are still being used to program one's behavior.

**LINEAR** Proceeding in a line or straight progression; having only one dimension.

**LOGIC** A particular method of reasoning.

**MANIPULATION** To manage or influence by artful or devious skill; to change to suit one's purpose or advantage.

**NEED** Something essential to the healthy life and growth of a person, as in "Babies *need* touching," "People *need* food and strokes." Also, that which is necessary according to the stage of development.

**POSITION** A fixed, psychological attitude.

**PROBLEM SOLVING** The process of finding solutions for problems or conflicts.

## GLOSSARY

**PROTECTION**  Setting up situations for safety, first by preventing trouble whenever possible and then by having effective ways of dealing with problems when they arise.

**PSYCHIC ENERGY**  The energy of the human soul or mind.

**REGRESSION**  The process of returning to earlier stages of development, using only the physical, mental and emotional systems then available in order to resolve developmental problems.

**REPARENTING**  The use of regression to replace early parental programs with new and healthy parental experiences.

**REPROGRAMMING**  The process of transforming an archaic ego state or program.

**RESISTANCE**  To fight against or withstand the effect of; a way of protecting oneself from an experience one feels is threatening.

**SCRIPT**  An unconscious life plan based on decisions made during childhood and reinforced by parents, like the written text of a play, as used in Transactional Analysis.

**STAGE**  A stable portion of the developmental cycle having its own needs, processes and distinctive characteristics. Also, a scene of action in the cycle of life; the platform upon which the primal theater of life is enacted.

**STRAIGHT**  Relating directly, without ulterior motives, in contrast to engaging in *games*.

**STROKE**  A unit of recognition such as a touch, a greeting or a kick.

**STRUCTURE**  Organized elements of experience constructed to serve as models for doing things.

**SUSTAINING SYSTEMS** Those body systems without which life cannot continue, e.g., respiratory, digestive, circulatory, eliminative and immunological.

**SYMBIOSIS** A transactional relationship which is characterized by sharing of the functions of feeling, thinking and doing between two or more people.

**TRANSACTION** An exchange of strokes consisting of a stimulus from one person and a response from another.

**TRANSACTIONAL ANALYSIS** A system of social psychiatry that provides methods of identifying what goes on between people; a form of psychotherapy; a complete theory of personality.

**TRANSFORMATION** Reprogramming past, painful experiences, replacing them with new, constructive ones.

**TRAUMA** A startling experience that has a lasting effect on mental life.

# About the Author

**PAMELA LEVIN, RN,** is an award—winning author and world—renowned innovator in the fields of physical and emotional health and healing.

She is a graduate of the University Of Illinois, and studied Transactional Analysis (TA) with its founder, Eric Berne. She was the first nurse and the first woman to be awarded Clinical Membership then Teaching Membership in its international organization. She has also completed over 400 post—graduate hours in advanced clinical nutrition, herbology and women's health.

For her pioneering work on the cyclic process of life, she received the Eric Berne Memorial Scientific Award from the members of the International Transactional Analysis Association. Her public speaking career includes both professional and lay audiences in ten countries on four continents.

Her articles and books have been translated into ten languages and have sold over 100,000 copies worldwide. They are based on the processes of healing she found to work for herself and her clients, and include:

*Cycles of Power: A User's Guide to the Seven Seasons of Life,*

# THE CYCLE OF LIFE

*Perfect Bones: A Six—Point Plan for Healthy Bones,* and
*The Female Hormone Journey: Lifetime Care of Your Hormones.*

For nearly forty years, she maintained a private practice in Northern California.

She is the mother of two children and grandmother of two.

# Acknowledgments

Eric Berne, who especially liked irreverent nurses; Claude Steiner, who made a challenge I could not refuse; the late Jacqui Schiff, who encouraged me to think *and* have needs; Ken Rashid, MD, for his powerful support and protection; my adventurous co—transformers and caretakers, who would rather live courageously than die in each moment; Laurie and Jon Weiss, who recognized significance in this material and provided their direct encouragements; Steve Karpman, who insisted that the material be written for all to share; Virginia Hilliker, who supported this risk—taking with her life and limb, who ate, slept and drank the theoretical constructs to assure their validity; my many new parents, who loved and nurtured me from birth to present and back again; Joan Menninger, who applied this material to the process of creative writing and then applied all that to me in loving form; Lloyd Linford and Jean Peters, who never failed support from the time of its conception on through labor and birth; the late Joe Concannon, my Clinical and Teaching sponsor, who never lost faith in my abilities, and so proved there really is a Santa Claus; Muriel James, the late Margaret Northcott, Peggy Love Tusler, Sheila Regan Coin, Emily Ruppert, Helen Colton, Pat Crossman and Peggy Cogswell for being

## The Cycle of Life

strong, competent and supportive women; Carla Haimowitz and Robert Mehler for their invaluable opinions, especially about this manuscript; Eleanor Regan, for her Herculean efforts, Zen typing skills and kind opinions; Loni Baur for her clarity and intelligent guidance with the second edition; Muriel Chapman, DO, Jim Yensan, Shoshana Swartz and Jason Zimmet for their invaluable work with bodies, mine in particular; Gail and Harold Nordeman for clear structure, complete commitment and loving constancy.

The talents and generosity of the following people were crucial to the development, shaping and completion of this book: Jean Caldwell, for her skillful assistance with computerizing the text; Lee Mothes for his ongoing artistic support through every edition; and Sandy Peters of ROP Business School in Ukiah, CA, for her help and support with designing the text. My manuscript readers were so generous with their time and opinions: Sunny Mehler, Layne Hackett, Eric and Kathy Landheer, Karen Miller, Jan Elliott, Felipe Garcia, Julia Mast, Bill Hallahan, Robin Fryer. My literary consultant, Diane Eble, of Words to Profit, provided her expertise and support all the way through. And to my fantastic and dedicated editors, a special debt of gratitude: Denise Maclachlan—Olling and Ronilyn McDonald.

# Notes

[1] Since that time a wealth of information has been gathered by a variety of health professionals on life in the womb and the effects of prenatal life on that after birth. For example, see Thomas Verney, MD with John Kelly, *The Secret Life of the Unborn Child,* Summit Books, USA, and Collins, Canada, 1981. Also see the Association for Pre— and Perinatal Psychology and Health, APPPAH www.birth psychology.com

[2] See *De 7 Keer Van Lammitie Pammetie (The Seven Stages of Lamiken Pammikin)* by Gode—Liva Willems, Uitegeverji Infodok, Belgium, Netherlands. 1989.

[3] *Self—Esteem: A Family Affair,* by Jean Clarke, Winston Press, Minnesota, 1998, is based on the developmental stages and messages presented in *Becoming the Way We Are.* Rokelle Lerner's *Daily Affirmations for Adult Children of Alcoholics,* Health Communications, Inc., Florida, 1996, used the developmental affirmations presented originally in *Becoming the Way We Are.*

[4] C. Annete Bodmer founded Affirmation Enterprises and wrote *The Gift of Affirmation*, Affirmation Enterprises, Savage, Minnesota, 1985.

[5] See John Bradshaw's *Homecoming: Reclaiming and Championing Your Inner Child,* Bantam Books, New York, 1990.

[6] The cycle was used as the basic text for the course "Theories of Human Development." Its students were Native peoples who spoke their Amerindian language and used French as a second language. By now the material had been presented in *Cycles of Power: A User's Guide to the Seasons of Life.*, 1980. From that the Canadian governmental translation service produced this first French version in 1983. It was then picked up by InterEditions, Paris (now Dunod) and has been in continuous publication since 1986.

[7] Osteopath Alexander Rupertini elaborates on the correlations between the patterns of our solar system and the patterns of our lives in *Cycles of Becoming: The Planetary Pattern of Growth*, CRCS Publications, Sebastapol, 1978.

[8] For a collection of spiral images as a mystical or cosmic symbol, including Stone Age art, Chinese symbols, Celtic crosses, Maori tattoos, Islamic arabesques and more, see Jill Purce's *The Mystic Spiral: Journey of the Soul*, Thames and Hudson, New York 1974. For the sym-

# NOTES

bols themselves along with their interpretations, see *Symbols —— Encyclopedia of Western Signs and Ideograms* by Carl G Liungman, HME Publishing, Lidingö, Sweden, 1998; or see http://www.symbols.com/encyclopedia/14/1414.html

[9] Jose Arguelles presents detailed holonomic maps of this spiral staircase in *Earth Ascending: An Illustrated Treatise on the Law Governing Whole Systems*, Shambhala Books, Boulder, Co. 1984.

[10] This pattern as it occurs in DNA was described in detail by Ruth Moore in *The Coil of Life: The Story of the Great Discoveries in the Life Sciences*, Alfred A. Knopf, New York, 1967.

[11] Edward R. Dewey, "The Case for Cycles" in *Cycles* Magazine 18, 1967, p. 162. For information on how cycles impact everything from the latest corn crop to the stock market, contact The Foundation for the Study of Cycles, Inc., 2929 Coors Blvd. NW Suite 307, Albuquerque, NM 87120 USA. Or see http://www.foundationforthestudyof cycles.org.

[12] Author Matila Ghyka asks if there is a natural aesthetic that corresponds to a universal order in *The Geometry of Art and Life,* Dover Edition, New York, 1977.

## The Cycle of Life

[13] The lyrics to "The Circle Game" were written by Joni Mitchell, copyright 1966 by Sequomb Publishing Corporation, quoted here with permission.

[14] This summation of the fractal nature of turbulence was written by British physicist and psychologist Lewis F. Richardson, as quoted in *Chaos: Making a New Science* by James Gleick, Penguin Books, 1987, p. 119. The poem condenses Richardson's 1920 paper "The supply of energy from and to Atmospheric Eddies."

[15] This principle is beautifully elaborated and illustrated in Gyorgy Doczi's *The Power of Limits; Proportional Harmonies in Nature, Art & Architecture*, Shambhala Publications, Boulder, 1981.

[16] See "A History of the Golden Mean/ Section/ Ratio/ Divine Proportion and Phi" at http://jwilson.coe.uga.edu/EMT668/EMAT6680.2000/Obara/Emat6690/Golden%20Ratio/golden.html

[17] This information is beautifully elaborated in Jacob Bronowski's television series and book chapter entitled *"The Long Childhood"* in *The Ascent of Man*, Little Brown & Co; Boston, 1974.

[18] For a presentation of the science behind the evolution of intelligence, see Carlos Sagan, *The Dragons of Eden: Speculations on the Evolution of Human Intelligence*, Ballantine Books, New York, 1986.

# NOTES

[19] Genesis, Chapter 1, Verses 1—31, King James Version of the Holy Bible.

[20] For an excellent presentation of the scientific discoveries behind this information, see Daniel Goleman's *Social Intelligence: The New Science of Human Relationships,* Bantam Books, New York, 2006.

[21] For material on scripts presented in detail, see Eric Berne's *What Do You Say After You Say Hello?*, Grove Press, New York, 1972; Claude Steiner's *Scripts People Live,* Grove Press, New York, 1974 and Muriel James and Dorothy Jongeward's *Born to Win,* Addison—Wesley, Boston, 1971.

[22] The relationship of the stress mechanism to exploratory dynamics was pointed out in a personal communication by Gracia Cass, R.N. and Paul Cass.

[23] Karpman, Steven. "Options," *Transactional Analysis Journal,* Vol. 1, No. 1, pp. 79—87, January 1971.

[24] Goulding, Robert. "New Directions in Transactional Analysis: Creating an Environment for Redecision and Change," a chapter in *Progress in Group and Family Therapy*, Brunner/Mazel, 1972.

[25] This work is reported in *The Evolutionary Neuroethology of Paul Maclean: Convergences and Frontiers* with contributions by Gerald A. Cory Jr., Russell Gardner Jr., editors, Praeger Publishers, Westport, Connecticut. 2002.

[26] Berne, Eric. *Transactional Analysis in Psychotherapy.* Grove Press, New York, 1961.

[27] This description of what is exchanged in stroking was used by Robert Bly to describe what the father gives the son, in *Iron John, A Book About Men,* Addison—Wesley, San Francisco, 1990, p 93.

[28] For further information on stroking, an excellent book is Montagu, Ashley. *Touching.* Harper & Row, New York, 1971.

[29] A thorough exposition of transactional games is contained in Berne, Eric. *Games People Play.* Grove Press, New York, 1971. For the developmental descriptions of games, see Levin, Pamela, *Cycles of Power: A User's Guide to the Seasons of Life,* The Nourishing Company, originally published 1980.

[30] Schiff, Aaron Wolfe and Schiff, Jacqui. "Passivity," *Transactional Analysis Journal,* Vol 1, No. 1, pp. 78—89, January, 1971.

# NOTES

[31] These basic three positions in all games were defined and elaborated in 1968 by Stephen Karpman, MD, in "Fairy Tales and Script Drama Analysis," *Transactional Analysis Bulletin*, Vol. 6, No. 26, pp. 39—43.

[32] This predicament is described by Robert Bly in *Iron Joh: A Book About Men*, Addison—Wesley, San Francisco, 1990, p. 45.

[33] See: Steiner, Claude. *Games Alcoholics Play*. Grove Press, New York, 1971; and Berne, Eric. *What Do You Say After You Say Hello?*, Grove Press, New York, 1971.

[34] For a presentation of what kinds of solutions people discovered as they underwent this process, see *Cycles of Power: A User's Guide to the Seasons of Life* by Pamela Levin, The Nourishing Company, Ukiah, California,1980. This was later elaborated by John Bradshaw in *Homecoming:, Reclaiming and Championing Your Inner Child*, Bantam Books, New York, 1990.

[35] For a thorough treatment of this subject, see *The Biology of Belief: Unleashing The Power Of Consciousness, Matter And Miracles,* by Bruce H. Lipton, Mountain of Love/Elite Books, Santa Rosa, California, 2005, or visit his website at www.BruceLipton.com. For a series of interviews on film, see *What the Bleep Do We Know?*

[36] English, Fanita. "Episcript and the Hot Potato Game," *Transactional Analysis Journal,* Vol. 8, No. 33, 1969.

[37] Levin, Pamela. "Think Structure for Feeling Fine Faster," *Transactional Analysis Journal,* Vol. 3, No. 1, pp. 38—39, January 1973.

[38] Clarke, J. I. Affirmation Structure, Personal Communication, 1980.

[39] Crossman, Patricia. "Permission and Protection," *Transactional Analysis Journal,* Vol. 5, No. 19, July, 1966.

[40] Berne, Eric. *Principles of Group Treatment.* Oxford University Press, New York, 1966.

[41] This process is adapted from one developed by the staff of a five—day experiential workshop called *Experiencing Enough Training,* Pamela Levin, RN, Elaine Childs—Gowell, RN, PhD, Gail Nordeman, RN, CTM and Harold Nordeman.

[42] For another view of programming and reprogramming experiences, see: John Lilly's *The Center of the Cyclone.* Julian Press, Inc., New York, 1972.

## NOTES

[43] William Wordsworth, "Ode: Intimations of Immortality from Recollections of Early Childhood". (ll. 63–67). *The Poems; Vol. 1* John O. Hayden, ed. Penguin Books, New York, 1977, repr. 1990.

[44] Corinthians 3, 16. *The Holy Bible, Hofman Pronouncing Edition, King James Version*, p. 1071.

How to be in touch:

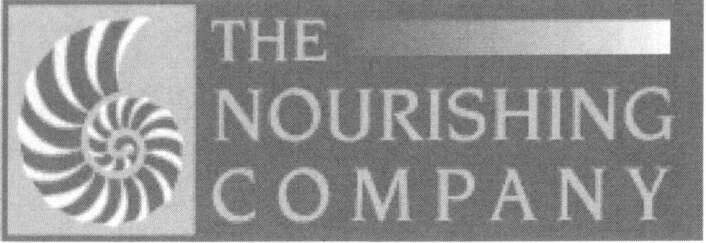

Go to *nourishingcompany*.com
for free articles that address the cycle and its phases.
You can also purchase additional copies of this and other books.

Register your book at **nourishingcompany.com**
so you can receive free updates on how to deal with
the challenges of living in nature's design.

While there, click "contact us" to share how you're putting nature's
design to work in your life. Yours may be a story
included in updates and news.

Or ask a question.
Yours may be one of the frequently asked questions
Pamela answers about being a grown-up on this cyclic path of life.

*THE NOURISHING COMPANY*
P.O. Box 1429
Ukiah,
Ca.
95482
*nourishingcompany.com*

THE NOURISHING COMPANY

How to be in touch:

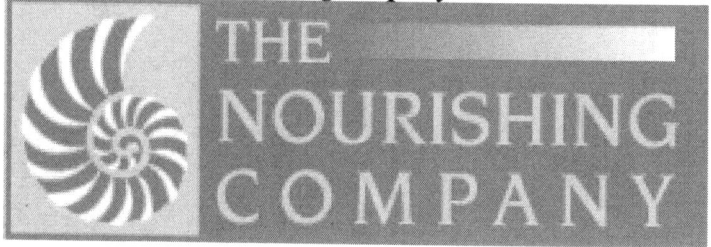

Go to *nourishingcompany*.com
for free articles that address the cycle and its phases.
You can also purchase additional copies of this and other books.

Register your book at **nourishingcompany.com**
so you can receive free updates on how to deal with
the challenges of living in nature's design.

While there, click "contact us" to share how you're putting nature's
design to work in your life. Yours may be a story
included in updates and news.

Or ask a question.
Yours may be one of the frequently asked questions
Pamela answers about being a grown-up on this cyclic path of life.

*THE NOURISHING COMPANY*
P.O. Box 1429
Ukiah,
Ca.
95482
*nourishingcompany.com*

**THE NOURISHING COMPANY**

How to be in touch:

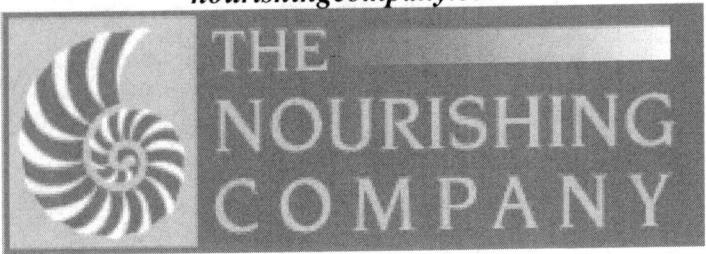

Go to *nourishingcompany*.com
for free articles that address the cycle and its phases.
You can also purchase additional copies of this and other books.

Register your book at **nourishingcompany.com**
so you can receive free updates on how to deal with
the challenges of living in nature's design.

While there, click "contact us" to share how you're putting nature's
design to work in your life. Yours may be a story
included in updates and news.

Or ask a question.
Yours may be one of the frequently asked questions
Pamela answers about being a grown-up on this cyclic path of life.

*THE NOURISHING COMPANY*
P.O. Box 1429
Ukiah,
Ca.
95482
*nourishingcompany.com*

THE NOURISHING COMPANY

How to be in touch:

Go to *nourishingcompany*.com
for free articles that address the cycle and its phases.
You can also purchase additional copies of this and other books.

Register your book at **nourishingcompany.com**
so you can receive free updates on how to deal with
the challenges of living in nature's design.

While there, click "contact us" to share how you're putting nature's
design to work in your life. Yours may be a story
included in updates and news.

Or ask a question.
Yours may be one of the frequently asked questions
Pamela answers about being a grown-up on this cyclic path of life.

*THE NOURISHING COMPANY*
P.O. Box 1429
Ukiah,
Ca.
95482
*nourishingcompany.com*

**THE NOURISHING COMPANY**

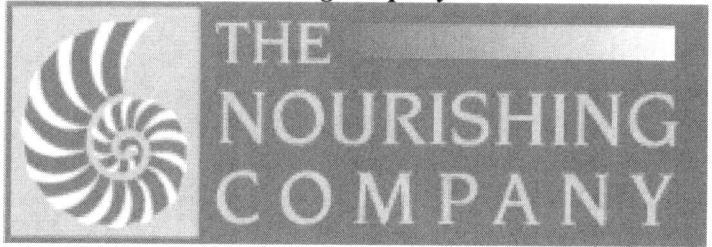